Pulmonary Pathophysiology for Pre-Clinical Students

Instructor Resources

How to Adopt This Book

This is an open textbook. That means that this book is freely available and you are welcome to use, adapt, and share this book with attribution according to the Creative Commons NonCommercial ShareAlike 4.0 (CC BY-NC-SA 4.0) license https://creativecommons.org/licenses/by-nc-sa/4.0. (Many, but not all images, illustrations, etc in this book are licensed under CC BY 4.0.)

Instructors reviewing, adopting, or adapting this textbook are encouraged to register at https://bit.ly/interest-preclinical. This assists the Open Education Initiative at Virginia Tech in assessing the impact of the book and allows us to more easily alert instructors of additional resources, features and opportunities.

Finding Additional Resources for Your Course

The main landing page for the book is https://pressbooks.lib.vt.edu/pulmonarypathophysiology.

This page includes:

- Links to multiple electronic versions of the textbook (PDF, ePub, HTML)
- Links to the instructor resource-sharing portal
- Link to errata document (report errors at https://bit.ly/feedback-preclinical)
- Links to other books within this series

Sharing Resources You've Created

Have you created any supplementary materials for use with Cardiovascular Pathophysiology for Pre-Clinical Students such as presentation slides, activities, test items, or a question bank? If so, please consider sharing your materials related to this open textbook. Please tell us about resources you wish to share by using this form: https://bit.ly/interest-preclinical or by directly sharing resources under an open license to the public-facing instructor sharing portal https://www.oercommons.org/groups/pre-clinical-resources/10133.

Customizing This Book

The Creative Commons Attribution NonCommercial-ShareAlike 4.0 license https://creativecommons.org/licenses/by-nc-sa/4.0/legalcode on this book allows customization and redistribution which is NonCommercial, that is "not primarily intended for or directed towards commercial advantage or monetary compensation."

Best practices for attribution are provided at https://wiki.creativecommons.org/wiki/ Best_practices_for_attribution.

This book is hosted in PDF and ePub in VTechWorks http://hdl.handle.net/10919/105411 in HTML in Pressbooks https://pressbooks.lib.vt.edu/pulmonarypathophysiology and via the LibreTexts platform https://med.libretexts.org/@go/page/34444. Pressbooks and LibreTexts platforms both offer customization/remixing.

Pulmonary Pathophysiology for Pre-Clinical Students

ANDREW BINKS

PDF AND EPUB FREE ONLINE AT: HTTPS://DOI.ORG/10.21061/PULMONARYPATHOPHYSIOLOGY

VTC | Virginia Tech Carilion School of Medicine

VIRGINIA TECH PUBLISHING

VIRGINIA TECH CARILION SCHOOL OF MEDICINE IN ASSOCIATION WITH VIRGINIA TECH PUBLISHING
ROANOKE, VA

Suggested citation: Binks, Andrew (2022). *Pulmonary Pathophysiology for Pre-Clinical Students*. Roanoke: Virginia Tech Carilion School of Medicine. https://doi.org/10.21061/pulmonarypathophysiology. Licensed with CC BY-NC-SA 4.0 https://creativecommons.org/licenses/by-nc-sa/4.0.

Publisher: This work is published by the Virginia Tech Carilion School of Medicine in association with Virginia Tech Publishing, a division of the University Libraries at Virginia Tech.

Virginia Tech Carilion School of Medicine 2 Riverside Circle Roanoke, VA 24016 USA

Virginia Tech Publishing University Libraries at Virginia Tech 560 Drillfield Drive Blacksburg, VA 24061 USA https://publishing.vt.edu publishing@vt.edu

This work is also distributed by LibreTexts, Davis, CA USA info@libretexts.org. Note: The LibreTexts version of this work at https://med.libretexts.org/@go/page/34444 may differ from this version.

Peer review: This book has undergone single-blind peer review by two external reviewers.

Accessibility statement: Virginia Tech Publishing is committed to making its publications accessible in accordance with the Americans with Disabilities Act of 1990. The Pressbooks (HTML) and ePub versions of this text are tagged structurally and include alternative text, which allows for machine readability.

Publication cataloging information:
Binks, Andrew, author
Pulmonary Pathophysiology for Pre-Clinical Students / Andrew Binks
Pages cm
ISBN 978-1-957213-08-8 (PDF)
ISBN 978-1-957213-11-8 (ePub)
ISBN 978-1-957213-10-1 (Pressbooks) https://pressbooks.lib.vt.edu/pulmonarypathophysiology
ISBN 978-1-957213-09-5 (Print)
URI (Universal Resource Identifier): http://hdl.handle.net/10919/105411
DOI https://doi.org/10.21061/pulmonarypathophysiology

1. Lungs -- Pathophysiology -- Textbooks
   Title RC756 .B56 2022

Disclaimer: The information in this textbook is intended for educational purposes only and is not meant to take the place of medical care, diagnoses, or services. Please see your healthcare provider about any health concerns.

Cover art: Lungs by iconmu via the Noun Project and Virus by Lars Meiertoberens via the Noun Project. CC BY 3.0.
Illustration and cover design: Kindred Grey

Contents

Introduction vii

About the Author ix

Instructor Resources x

1. The Obstructive Lung Diseases 1

Asthma 1

Chronic Obstructive Pulmonary Disease 8

Cystic Fibrosis 15

Bronchiectasis 19

2. Upper Airway Infections 25

The Common Cold 26

Rhinosinusitis 27

Pharyngitis 27

Viral Croup 27

Bacterial Infection of the Upper Airway 28

3. Lower Airway Infections 30

Acute Bronchitis 30

Infectious Bronchiolitis 31

Pneumonia 32

4. The Restrictive Lung Diseases 39

Basis of Restrictive Lung Disease 39

Forms of Interstitial Lung Disease 43

5. Acute Respiratory Distress Syndrome 54

Pathology of ARDS 54

Stages of ARDS 56

Systemic pathophysiology of ARDS 57

Clinical signs of ARDS 58

6. Lung Cancer 60

Squamous Cell 60

Adenocarcinoma 61

Large Cell 61

Small Cell 61

Clinical Signs 62

7. Pulmonary Embolism 64
Pathology of Pulmonary Embolism (PE) 64
Pathophysiology of PE 65
Clinical Signs of PE 66
8. Immunological Diseases of the Lung 67
Hypersensitivity Pneumonitis 69
Goodpasture's Syndrome 70
Systemic Diseases Affecting the Lung 71
Summary 74
9. Pleural Diseases 76
Pleurisy 76
Pleural Effusion 77
Pneumothorax 80

Introduction

Pulmonary Pathophysiology for Pre-Clinical Students is an undergraduate medical-level resource for foundational knowledge of pulmonary pathophysiology. This text is designed for a course pre-clinical undergraduate medical curriculum and it is aligned to USMLE(r) (United States Medical Licensing Examination) content guidelines. The text is meant to provide the essential information in a concise format that would allow learner preparation to engage in an active classroom. Clinical correlates and additional application of content is intended to be provided in the classroom experience. The text assumes that the students will have an understanding of basic pulmonary physiology that will be helpful to understand the content presented here. This resource should be assistive to the learner later in medical school and for exam preparation given the material is presented in a succinct manner, with a focus on high-yield concepts.

The 80+ page text was created specifically for use by pre-clinical students at Virginia Tech Carilion School of Medicine and was based on faculty experience and peer review to guide development and hone important topics.

Pulmonary Pathophysiology for Pre-Clinical Students is intended to address both necessary content and align with the preclerkship curricular needs. The utility of a flexible text can positively impact the learning environment and increase student engagement and performance. This text is made to be adaptable by using pieces and parts to suit students and inspire the addition of elements to this living resource.

Features of this Book

- Learning objectives are provided at the beginning of each subsection
- High resolution, color contrasting figures illustrate concepts, relationships, and processes throughout
- Summary tables display detailed information
- Accessibility features including structured heads and alternative-text provide access for readers accessing the work via a screen-reader

This resource was designed to fill a gap in undergraduate medical education (UME) and support preclerkship education in the content areas of basic science for medical education. Unlike traditional textbooks, the organization of this resource is driven by curricular structure, rather than subject area. As the format and design of UME differs across many programs, this resource is purposefully brief and flexible, allowing for rapid adaptation across programs. The resource is organized into small chapters that can be used to support student preparation in any arrangement. The sections are not intended to be all-inclusive, but rather primers for applied content delivery. In our curriculum, these topic areas are interwoven into problem-based and case based learning modalities. The cases and clinical correlates change regularly and having the flexibility of these short resources that can be applied to many scenarios across the pre-clinical years of our curriculum is beneficial.

Over the past twenty years, medical education has undergone a rapid curricular restructuring. This is in part due to recommendations of the Flexner report[1], coupled with the changes observed in millennial[2] and iGen learners. To accommodate the integration of additional core competencies, the majority of medical programs have moved away from discipline-based delivery and currently use some form of integrated curricular format.[3] This allows material to be presented in a more clinically realistic and pertinent format without the constraints of artificial discipline silos. This movement has had positive impacts on programmatic outcomes and student performance, but it has presented some challenges for curricular design, student engagement and educational resources.

Although contemporary medical curricula have moved to a cohesive, integrated format, the required textbooks for undergraduate medical education remain traditional and discipline-based. Use of small, independent chapters allows content to be delivered in a variety of curricular settings and support content integration and alignment.

A high volume of content, some of it lacking alignment with class sessions coupled with restrictions on student contact time imposed by accrediting bodies, means that faculty across the country are having to rethink preparation materials to facilitate efficient, focused learning experiences. This resource It is intended to provide learners with a high-level view of relevant topical areas that will be further elaborated on within the classroom setting. Unlike other traditional textbooks, it is not intended to include all content a learner would need about the relevant subject area but to function as a stepping stone towards mastery of the content.

As programs embrace the philosophy of student-directed learning embedded in adult learning theory, more simplified readily available resources will be essential to support this fast-paced learning of health professional educational programs. While there are many factors that can contribute to a student's lack of preparation, lengthy textbook resources for a single integrated classroom session have a significant negative impact. So while an integrated curricular model enhances many aspects of learning, it makes using traditional textbooks cumbersome and disjointed for students. This resource hopes to address this concern.

Finally, there is a wealth of "medical" content freely accessible online, and students can find themselves spending a significant amount of time trying to identify alternative resources that may—or may not—be appropriate. Faculty taking ownership to identify and adapt realistic materials for each session reduces the concern that students are finding misinformation through internet sources, and this project allows faculty to create a resource that harnesses the best attributes of many different formats into a product that best supports the learning environment. Otherwise, external online resources are also likely to contain extraneous content that is not aligned with the classroom learning objectives (akin to subject-based textbook chapters), so it can also reduce the perceived worth of preparation. If the integrated resource is generated correctly, concisely and accurately by the faculty, the students will gain trust, rely on the vetted resources and prepare for the active classroom.

References

1. Cooke M, Irby DM, Ph D, et al. American Medical Education 100 Years after the Flexner Report. 2006: 1339-1344.
2. Roberts DH, Newman LR, Schwartzstein RM. Twelve tips for facilitating Millennials' learning. Medical Teacher. 2012; 34: 274-278.
3. VanTassel-Baska J, Wood S. The integrated curriculum model (ICM). Learning and Individual Differences. 2010; 20(4): 345-357.

About the Author

Dr. Andrew Binks is a cardiopulmonary physiologist who gained his BSc (Hons) in Physiological Sciences at the University of Newcastle upon Tyne, then a MSc in Human and Applied Physiology from King's College, London. He returned to Newcastle to do his PhD and study the underlying physiological mechanisms of dyspnea, the cardinal symptom of cardiopulmonary disease. He continued investigating dyspnea at Harvard School of Public Health as a postdoctoral fellow and then as a research scientist. After seven years at Harvard, Andrew took his first faculty position at the University of New England where he taught cardiovascular and pulmonary physiology to health profession and medical students. He continued to teach medical students their heart and lung physiology after moving to the University of South Carolina's Medical School in Greenville where he also directed the school's heart and lung pathophysiology courses. Andrew currently teaches heart and lung physiology and pathophysiology at Virginia Tech Carilion School of Medicine, directs the heart and lung pathophysiology course and has also served as the departmental director of faculty development.

In his two decades of teaching medical physiology, Andrew has regularly drawn upon his dyspnea research experience to generate an active, clinically focused approach to medical education. This book is part of that approach and supports students preparing for class with the basic information with the intention to apply and contextualize that information in a guided case-based classroom experience.

Andrew has published numerous peer-reviewed research papers and book chapters about dyspnea and about contemporary medical education. He has also given keynote presentations, faculty workshops and international webinars to promote effective medical education for the modern adult learner.

Acknowledgments

Funding and In-Kind Support
Publication of this work is made possible in part through the support of VIVA (Virtual Library of Virginia), LibreTexts, the Open Education Initiative of the University Libraries at Virginia Tech, and Virginia Tech Publishing.

Peer Reviewers
Alex Atwood, Medical Resident
Michael North, Medical Resident

Editorial Team
Managing Editor: Anita Walz
Graphic Design and Editorial Assistance: Kindred Grey
Alternative Text: Andrew Binks

Special Thanks
Delmar Larson, Founder, LibreTexts
Christa Miller, Accessible Technologies, Virginia Tech

1. The Obstructive Lung Diseases

Learning objectives

- Use pathophysiological characteristics of asthma to distinguish it from other pulmonary disorders.
- Determine the likely cause of airway hyperreactivity from a patient history.
- Use the pathophysiological characteristics of chronic bronchitis and emphysema to distinguish them from other pulmonary disorders.
- Interpret the findings of a physical examination of a person with chronic obstructive pulmonary disease (COPD).
- Describe the pathophysiology of cystic fibrosis.
- Describe the pathological and clinical manifestations of cystic fibrosis.
- Learn the possible etiologies and pathophysiology of bronchiectasis.
- Distinguish the presence of bronchiectasis from patient history, exam, and radiography.

Asthma

Asthma is a commonly occurring member of the obstructive lung disorders and is distinguished by its acute, or episodic, nature. It affects between 5 and 7 percent of the U.S. population and is characterized by a hyperresponsive airway that shows episodic bronchoconstriction, inflammation, and elevated mucous secretion.

About half of asthma arises before ten years old, and about one-third of all cases have a genetic or familial component.

There are numerous underlying mechanisms of asthma (figure 1.1), and they may not be exclusive or independent within the same patient.

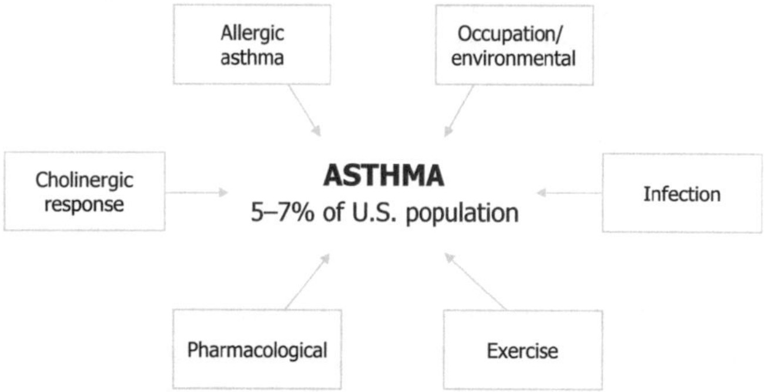

Figure 1.1: Forms and prevalence of asthma.

- **Allergic asthma:** (sometimes called atopic, or extrinsic, asthma) is probably the *most common* and thoroughly researched.
- **Cholinergic:** Because airways are under neural control, asthma can also be caused by failing autonomic reflexes.
- **Occupational/environmental:** Inhaled environmental substances, particularly those found in certain work places, can also sensitize airway responses.
- **Infection:** Triggering of inflammatory responses to infection can also produce or exacerbate an asthmatic response.

We will also look at how **exercise** and certain **pharmacological agents** can produce asthma.

<u>Allergenic asthma:</u> Most allergic asthma is caused by the presence of an excessive amount of **IgE** (the hallmark antibody of an allergy). Formation of an immune complex between the antigen and the overexpressed IgE results in binding to surface receptors on mast cells and basophilic granulocytes, of which there are plenty in the lung. The IgE receptor binding results in the release of a cocktail of proinflammatory and airway-active substances. Some of these, including **histamine** and **cytokines** that attract **eosinophils** and **neutrophils**, are stored in vesicles of mast cells shown in figure 1.2. Others are produced on demand, including **leukotrienes**, and are derivatives of **arachidonic acid** (we will return to this later).

The results of this cocktail's release are the hallmarks of asthma:

- contraction of smooth muscle in the airway, producing bronchoconstriction;
- microvascular leaking and congestion, producing airway wall edema; and
- increased airway secretion.

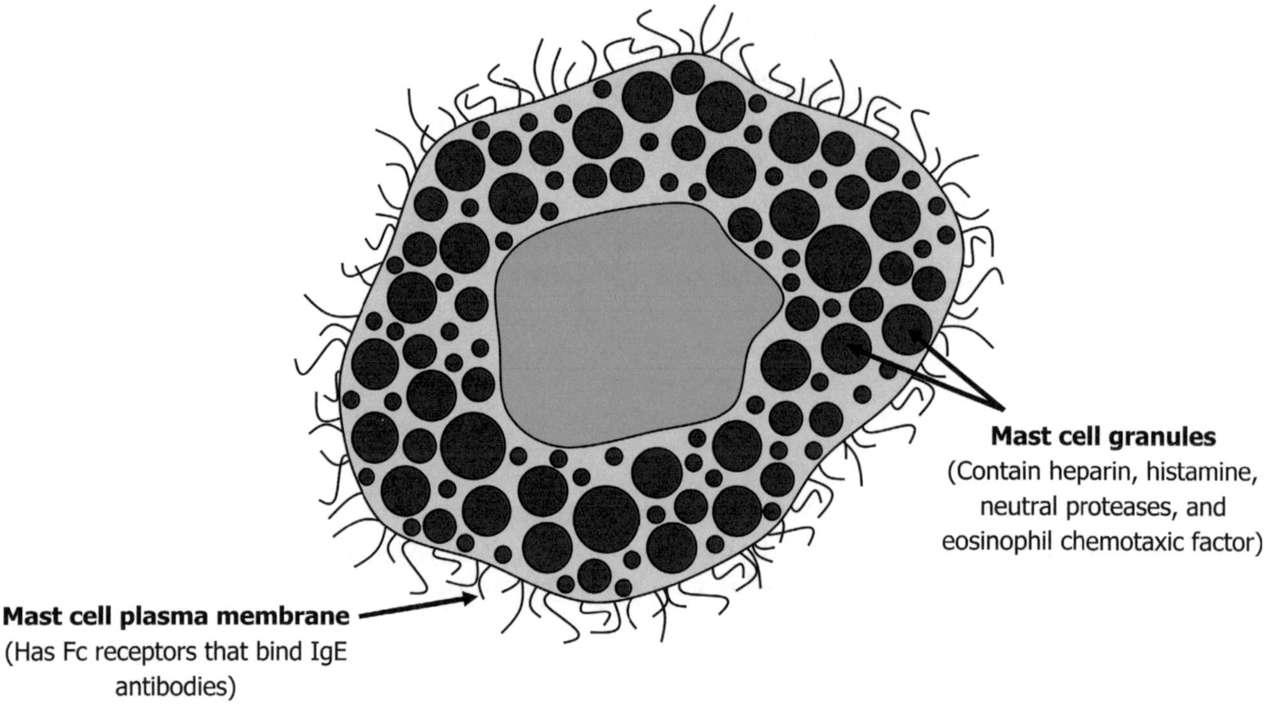

Figure 1.2: Example of a mast cell loaded with secretory granules.

The timeline from the exposure to the antigen to asthmatic response is not straightforward. A response may occur within minutes ("early response"), or hours later ("late response"). Some patients show only an early response, some only a late one, and some show both in a "dual" response. The late response may correspond to the arrival of leucocytes in response to the initial release of cytokines. It may also be due to a mild stimulus arriving later in an airway that was sensitized earlier.

<u>Cholinergic asthma:</u> Because it is open to the external environment, the airway has defensive, vagal reflexes (figure 1.3). An inappropriate exaggeration of some of these may lead to asthma. The basic reflex arch that ends with a cholinergic response begins with stimulation of airway irritant receptors in the epithelium. An afferent signal to the brainstem instigates an efferent signal to cause airway smooth muscle contraction and mucus secretion by glandular cells. The reflex also stimulates mast cells to release their cocktail, which includes histamine.

The released histamine stimulates the airway receptors, setting up the potential for a positive feedback loop and perpetuating the cycle of bronchoconstriction and secretion. The histamine also stimulates bronchoconstriction through its direct action on the smooth muscle as well as sensitizing the smooth muscle to further vagal stimulation. These processes are summarized in figure 1.3.

The cholinergic response may help produce an asthmatic response to another stimulus that normally would not have produced one (i.e., it may play a part in the hypersensitivity of the asthmatic airways). Likewise, the presence of an infection, particularly a viral infection, may place the airway in a proinflammatory state.

Neural airway control may also contribute to the high prevalence of nocturnal asthma, as during rest when the airways are predominantly under parasympathetic control. But other factors (summarized in figure 1.4) may contribute:

- Normal circadian fluctuations in epinephrine, cortisol, histamine, and other circulating factors may leave the airway more susceptible at night or the early morning.
- The normal suppression of the cough reflex may leave secretions in the airway and promote a proinflammatory state.
- The airway may also be demonstrating a late response to an exposure that happened earlier in the day.
- Being in the supine position promotes gastric reflux, which, while not necessarily causing aspiration, can induce oesphageal vagal reflexes that instigate the airway defensive reflexes we have just seen.

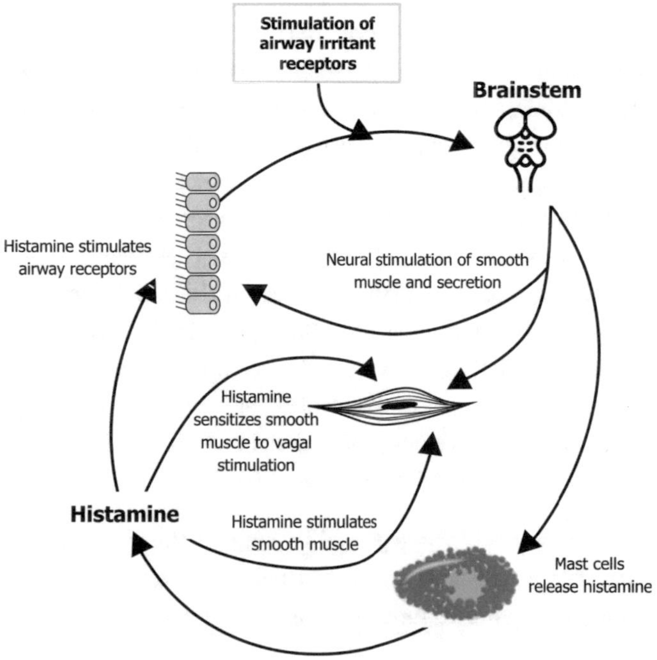

Figure 1.3: Vagal reflex of irritant airway receptors and the onset of asthma.

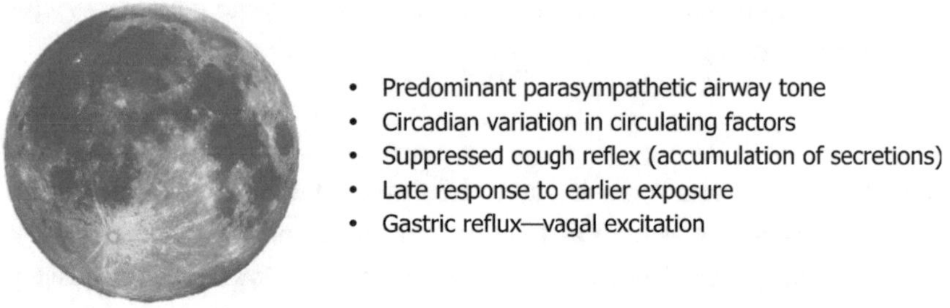

Figure 1.4: Factors promoting asthma at night.

Exercise-induced asthma: Although exercise is associated with increased airway caliber, it can also induce asthma. Increased airway flow to meet the increased metabolic demand of exercise results in loss of fluid and heat from airway surfaces. This leaves the peribronchial fluid in a hypertonic state and causes excitation of the irritant airway receptors, which leads to release of the mast cells' cocktail.

Exercise-induced asthma is more prevalent in cold (i.e. dry air) where water loss will be higher, so occurs more in sports such as cross-country skiing than swimming in a warm humid environment. Bronchoconstriction usually occurs when exercise stops—when the protective effect of sympathetic activity to the airway smooth muscles ceases.

Drug-induced asthma: There are several pharmaceutical and food products that can promote asthma, including tartrazine (a yellow food coloring) and sulfides used as food preservatives. Additionally, 10 to 20 percent of asthmatics are sensitive to aspirin.

Recall that some of the on-demand components of the mast cell's cocktail were derived from arachidonic acid. There are two pertinent pathways in which arachidonic acid is used: the lipoxygenase pathway and the cyclooxygenase pathway (figure 1.5). The first leads to the production of leukotrienes, which are potent bronchoconstrictors. The second leads to the production of prostaglandins and thromboxane. Normally the distribution of arachidonic acid down these pathways is balanced to meet demand. However, NSAIDS such as aspirin are COX 2 inhibitors and block the cyclooxygenase route, leaving more substrate for the lipoxygenase pathway and production of leukotrienes (figure 1.5) with their bronchoconstrictive effect.

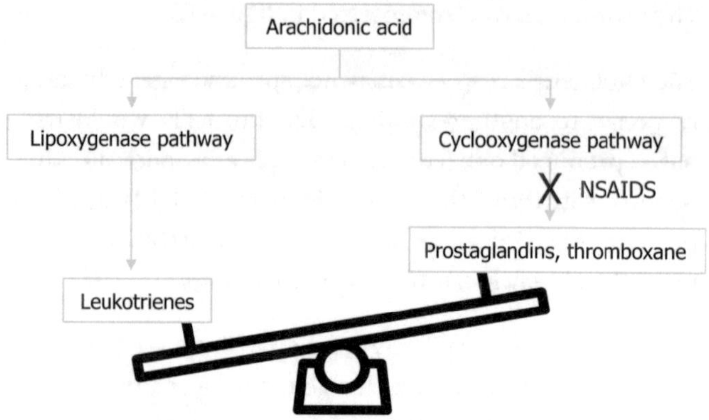

Figure 1.5: NSAIDS, including aspirin, shift metabolism of arachidonic acid toward bronchoconstrictive leukotrienes.

Environmental/occupational asthma: As the airway is open to the environment, it is susceptible to inhaled substances that can cause sensitization; there are over two hundred substances known to cause asthma, both organic and inorganic. Some common ones are listed below.

Chemical	Occurrence
Isocyanates	Polyurethane, plastics, varnish, spray paints
Trimellitic anhydride	Epoxy resins
Organic dust	Plants, grains, animal products

Table 1.1: Some of the most common environmental causes of asthma. Taking a pulmonary history should include asking about potential environmental exposures.

Determining whether airway hypersensitivity is due to environmental factors is complicated by widely varying latency periods. Short latency periods can be as brief as twenty-four hours and are associated with vapor or smoke exposure that does not cause an immunological response. Longer latency periods that may last years are more commonly associated with an immunological response to large particles that act like antigens.

The situation is further confused by occupation-related responses, which often cause the airway to become more sensitive to some of the other causes of asthma covered here. This makes the role of an environmental factor more difficult to determine.

Pathophysiology of Asthma

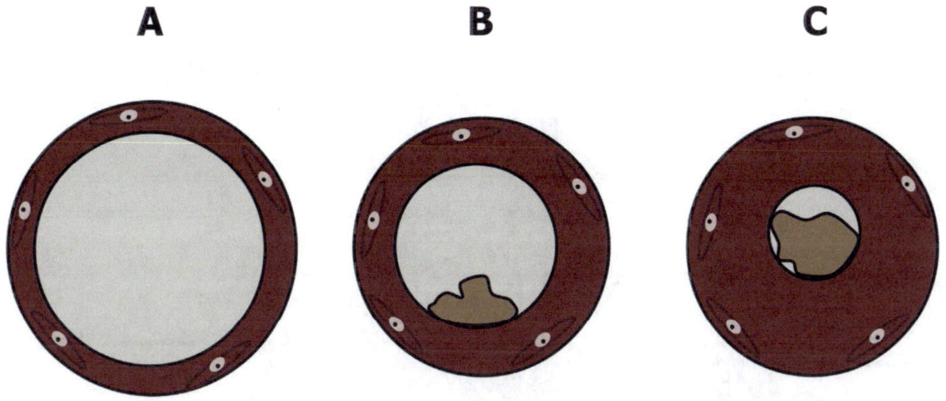

Figure 1.6: Illustrations of normal (A), mildly asthmatic (B), and severely asthmatic (C) airways.

With numerous and maybe concurrent mechanisms, what does asthma look like in the airway? The normal lumen of the airway has a relatively lower resistance, as depicted in panel A of figure 1.6, but in mild asthma the lumen is narrowed (thereby raising resistance to airflow) through swelling of the airway wall, contraction of airway smooth muscle, and blockage (or plugging) of the airway by increased mucus secretion (figure 1.6B). This worsens in more severe asthma until the lumen can be extremely narrow (figure 1.6C) or even completely blocked.

Other characteristics of asthma include the presence of eosinophillic that infiltrate into the airway walls. The eosinophil enzymes also leave a telltale sign: Charcot-Leyden crystals, as shown in the circled area of figure 1.7A.

The sputum of the asthmatic may also contain Curshman's spirals (figure 1.7B), which are casts of small bronchioles consisting of mucus and shed epithelial cells. However, Curshman's spirals are not exclusive to asthma.

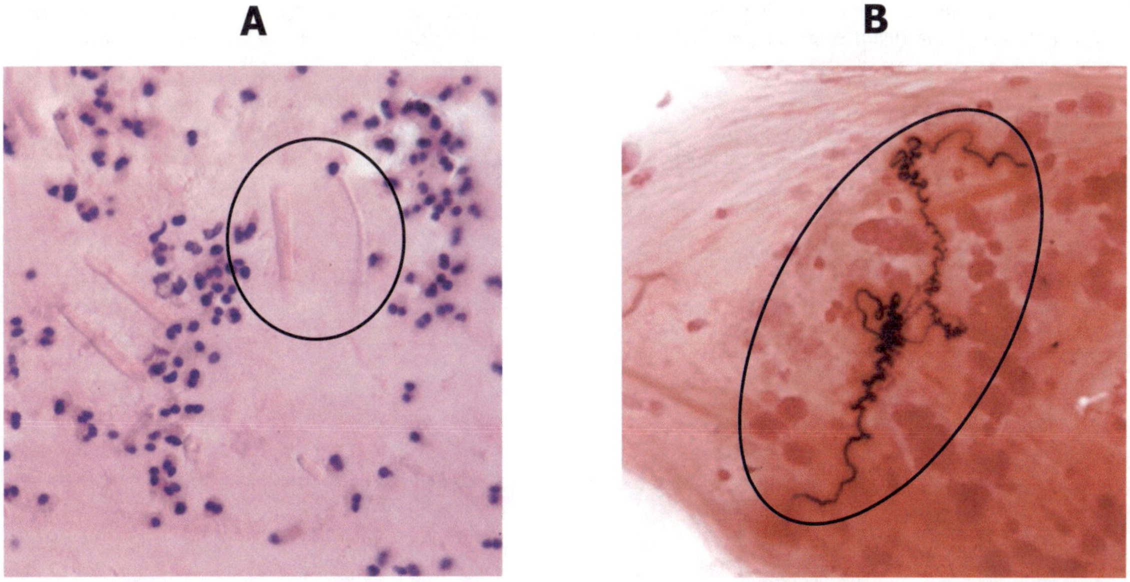

Figure 1.7: Histological signs of asthma: A = Charcot-Leyden crystals, B = Curshman's spirals.

With persistent asthma the airway undergoes remodeling (figure 1.8), with thickening of the airway wall and basement membrane, enlarged submucosal glands, and hypertrophy and hyperplasia of airway smooth muscle.

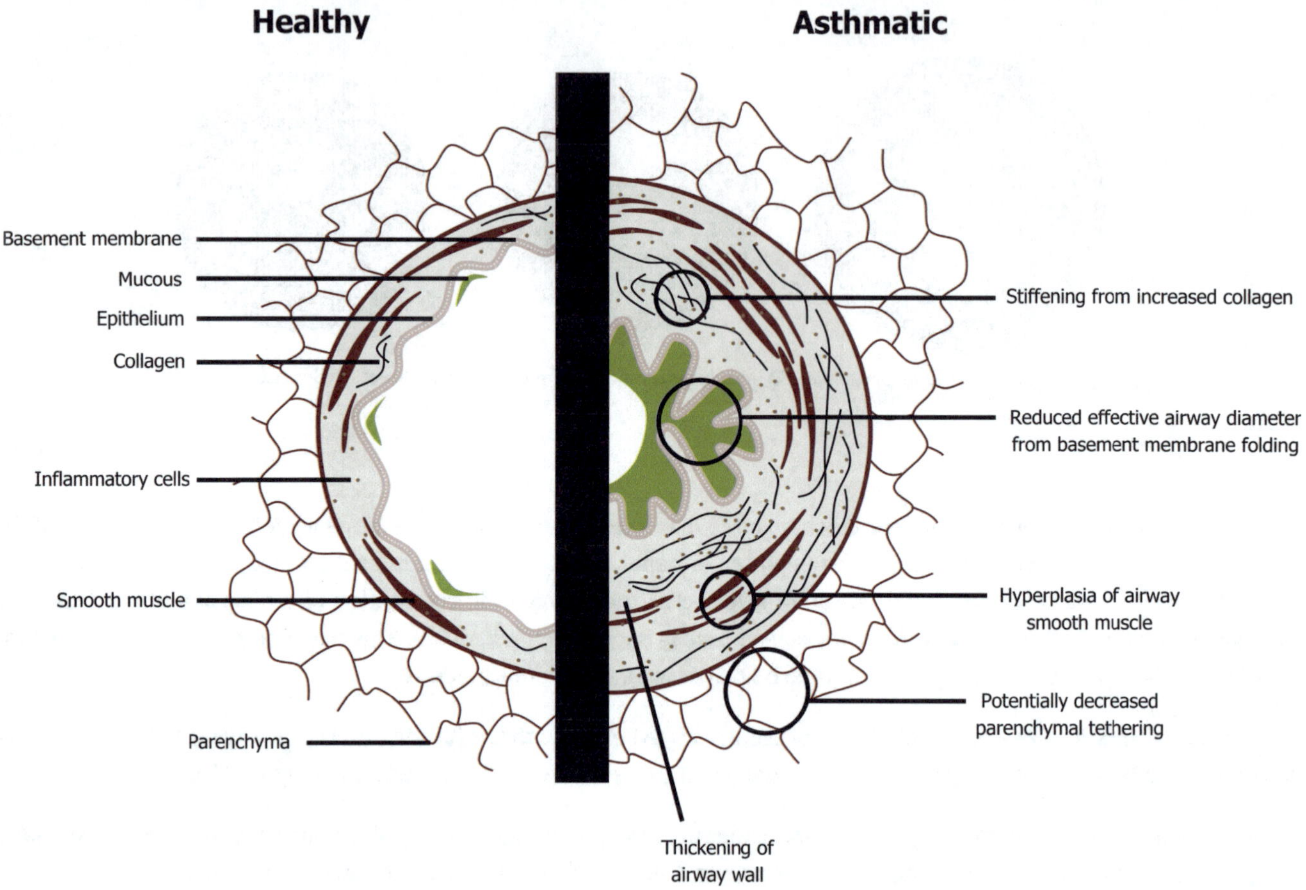

Figure 1.8: Components of airway remodeling in persistent asthma. The epithelium in asthma shows mucous hyperplasia and hypersecretion (gray), and significant basement membrane thickening. Smooth muscle volume is also increased in asthma.

Clinical Presentation of Asthma

One useful diagnostic element of asthma is its **episodic** or **acute** behavior. However, as patients may be asymptomatic between attacks, the severity of asthma can be difficult to determine without performing bronchial challenge tests.

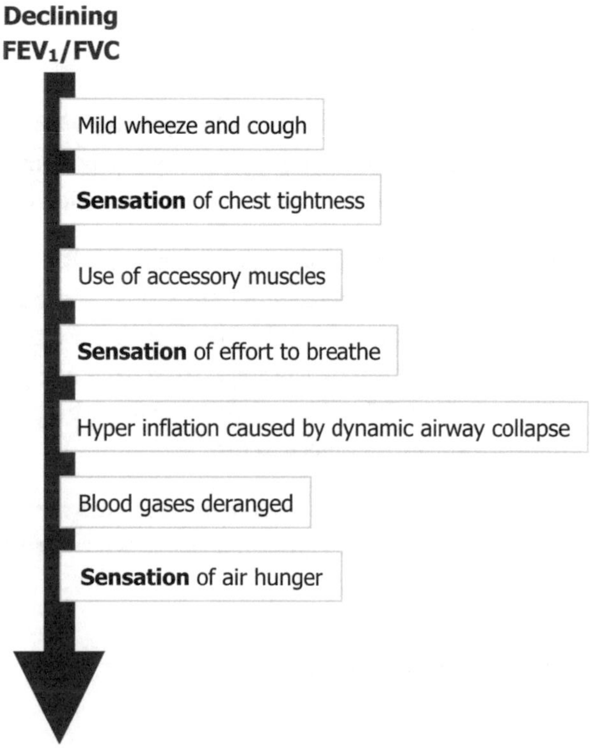

Figure 1.9: The progression of an asthma "attack."

The characteristic signs of asthma progress and vary with declining FEV_1 (summarized in figure 1.9). Most attacks start with mild wheezing and coughing, which progress with the severity of attack. The location and form of sensations vary between patients, but most asthmatics complain of chest tightness. This sensation is more commonly reported by asthmatics than other pulmonary patients, so it is a useful diagnostic sign.

As airway resistance increases, the accessory muscles are deployed to maintain sufficient airflow through the narrowing airways, and the patient experiences an increased effort to breathe. Increased expiratory efforts produce dynamic airway collapse and lead to hyperinflation. Further decreases in airway caliber result in insufficient alveolar ventilation and deranged blood gases. The sensation reported at this point is air hunger. Once the patient is severely bronchoconstricted, delivery of inhaled therapies is much more difficult, and mechanical ventilation to support the respiratory muscles becomes complicated. Other signs present during a severe attack are raised heart (tachycardia) and breathing (tachypnea) rates as well as a paradoxical pulse (i.e., a rise in blood pressure during expiration).

The typical chest x-ray of an asthmatic (figure 1.10) shows hyperlucent lung fields, evidence of hyperinflation and peribronchial infiltrate, and perhaps areas of atelectasis. However, the chest x-ray is not particularly effective at distinguishing asthma from some other obstructive disorders.

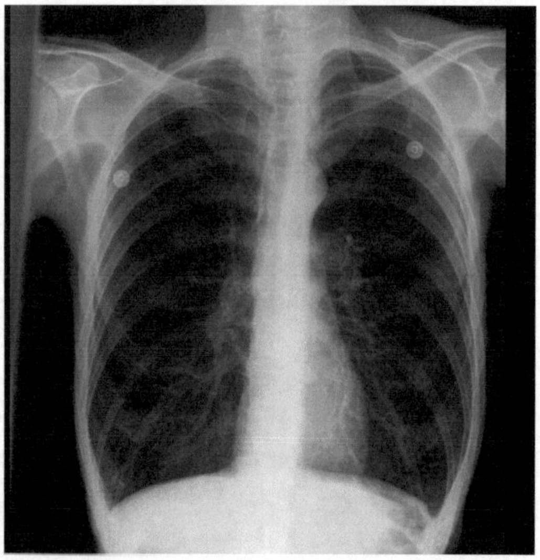

Figure 1.10: Typical chest x-ray of an asthmatic patient showing hyperlucent fields and hyperinflation. Notice the flattened diaphragm and the number of ribs that are visible; more than six anterior ribs or ten posterior ribs being visible is indicative of hyperinflation.

Chronic Obstructive Pulmonary Disease

Chronic obstructive pulmonary disease, or COPD, actually covers two obstructive disorders—chronic bronchitis and emphysema.

Although chronic bronchitis and emphysema have different underlying pathologies, they frequently have the same root cause and are often found together in a patient. In brief, chronic bronchitis is associated with an increase in mucus production, while emphysema involves disruption of the lung structure.

The relative role of chronic bronchitis in COPD has diminished since the Clean Air Act reduced atmospheric sulphur dioxide, but with 90 percent of COPD caused by cigarette smoking there is still plenty of bronchitis and emphysema to treat—at enormous cost to the health system from over eight million hospitalizations a year that are mostly paid for by Medicare. The COPD patient tends to be older and poorer and will likely have comorbidities, the most common of which is hypertension. What is perhaps more disturbing is that of the most common causes of death, COPD is the only one whose incidence continues to rise.

We will now look at the underlying mechanisms of COPD. Despite the fact it is usually composed of some elements of both chronic bronchitis and emphysema, we will deal with each separately for the sake of simplicity.

Chronic Bronchitis

Chronic bronchitis is clinically defined as a persistent and productive cough that lasts for at least three months per year for two consecutive years.

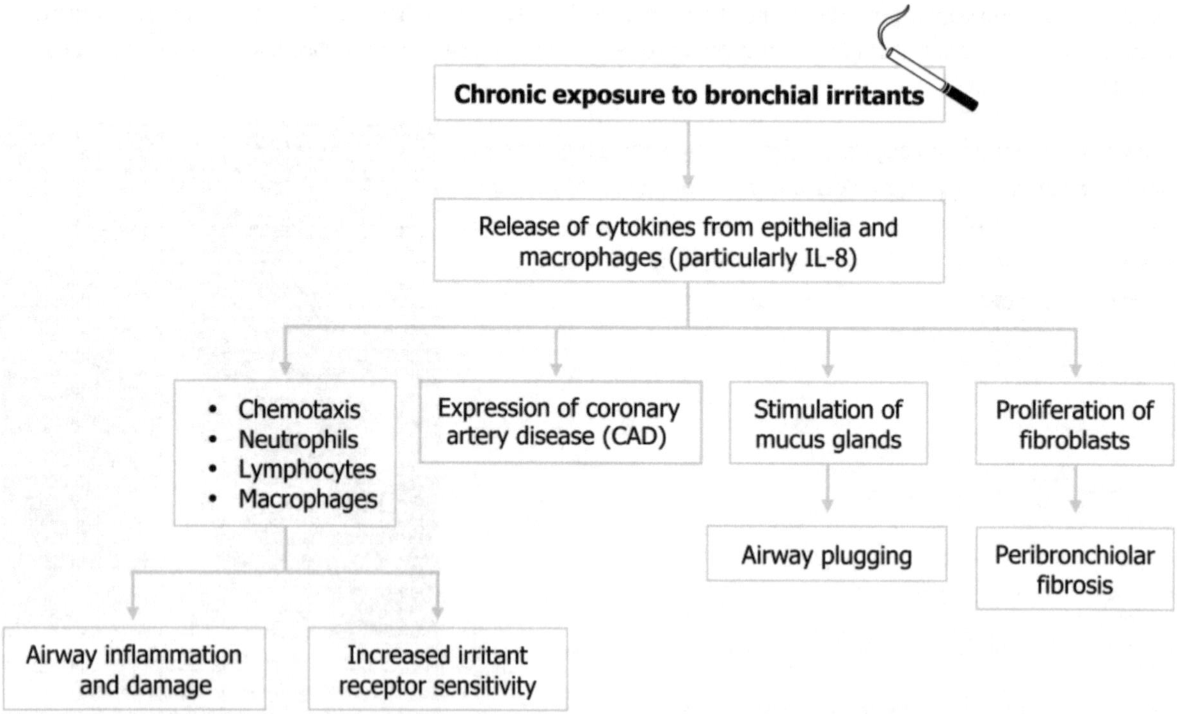

Figure 1.11: Pathophysiology of chronic bronchitis.

Chronic bronchitis arises from chronic exposure to bronchial irritants, the most common of which is tobacco smoke. These irritants initiate the release of cytokines from airway epithelial cells and macrophages that result in a cascade of responses (summarized in figure 1.11).

Neutrophils, lymphocytes, and macrophages are attracted to the irritated airway, and their presence is maintained through increased expression of cell adhesion molecules on the airway walls. These immune cells lead to acute airway wall inflammation that narrows the airway, and if chronic, can lead to tissue damage. The cytokines released by these cells also sensitize airway irritant receptors, which exacerbates the response to future irritant exposure.

Mucus production increases, and the glands themselves may also release cytokines that further exacerbate the inflammatory response. The mucus also contributes to airway narrowing, and mucus plugs may form that completely block bronchioles.

Mesenchymal cells transition into fibroblasts as part of the inflammatory response, and their chronic presence leads to the deposition of fibrotic tissue.

Collectively these responses to the irritants result in a narrowed airway that is **(1) hypersensitive, (2) fibrosed, and (3) blocked** by excessive secretions.

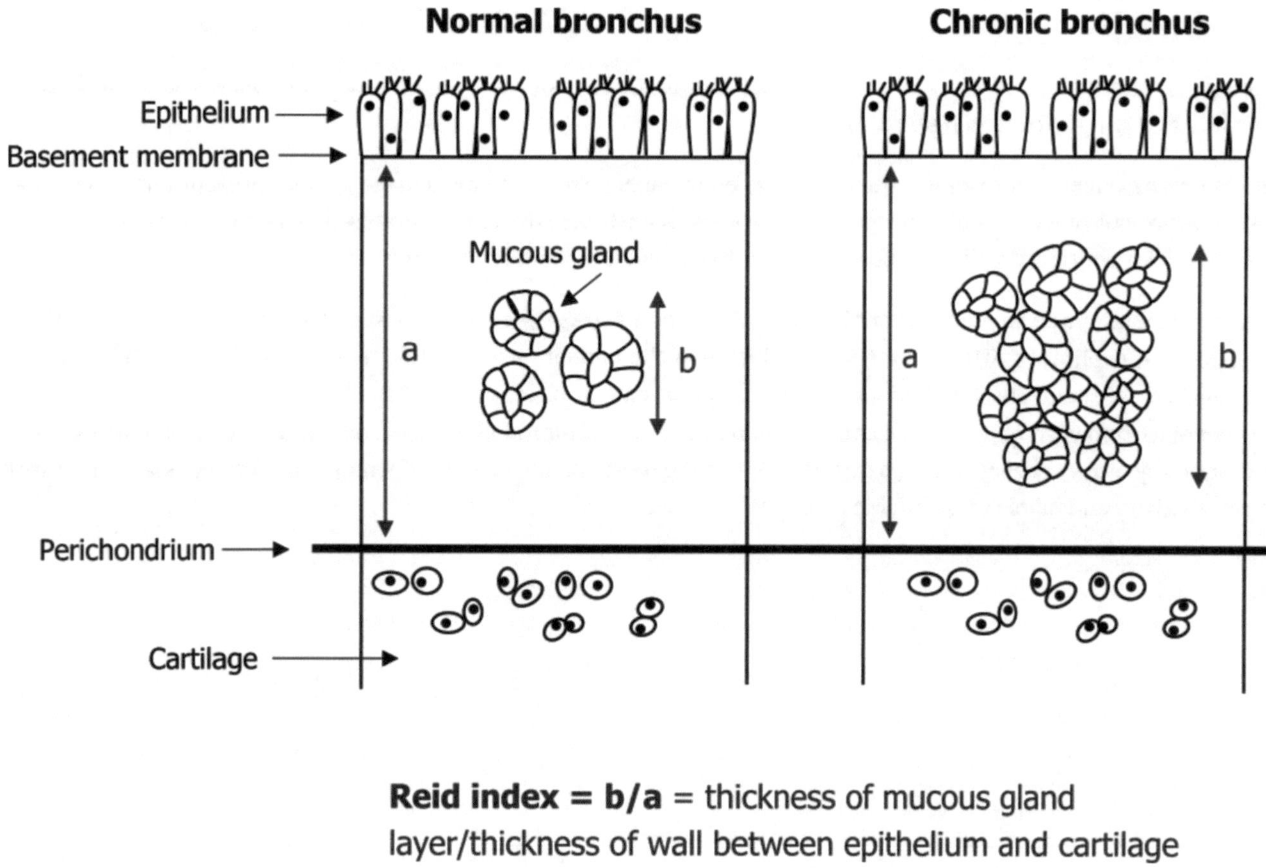

Figure 1.12: The Reid index compares the width of mucus glands to the width of the submucosal layer of airways.

Continued exposure to irritants leads to other chronic changes beyond fibrosis. With excessive stimulation, the size and number of mucus glands increases. The size of mucosal glands is used as a diagnostic test, and the Reid index describes what proportion of the submucosa is spanned by a gland—in the normal airway a normal gland spans less than 40 percent of the submucosa's depth, but in chronic bronchitis this exceeds 50 percent (figure 1.12).

In conjunction with an increased mucus production capacity, the airway has a reduced mucus clearance capability with airway remodeling, including squamous metaplasia replacing normal ciliated columnar epithelium (figure 1.13). The mucus escalator is also compromised by a decline in function of the remaining cilia with exposure to cigarette smoke.

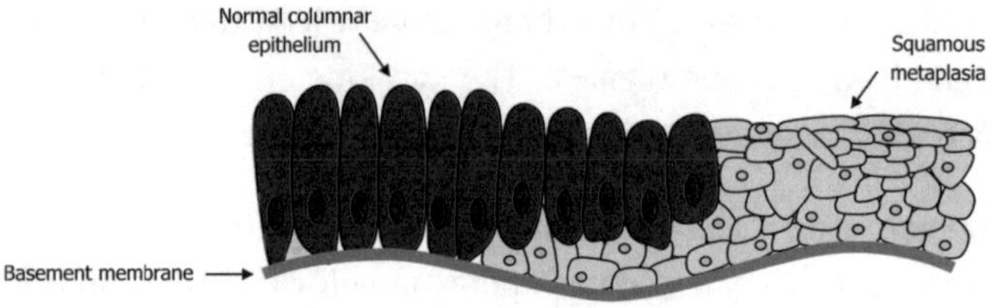

Figure 1.13: Prolonged irritant exposure can lead to airway remodeling with loss of normal ciliated epithelium.

These changes result in an airway that produces more mucus and is less capable of removing it. The static mucus not only causes airway plugging, but can also promote infections that lead to episodic and characteristic exacerbation of COPD symptoms.

Clinical Presentation of Chronic Bronchitis

The signs and symptoms of chronic bronchitis depend on the level of airway obstruction and the consequent decline in lung function (summarized in figure 1.14).

As with many pulmonary diseases, the onset can be insidious. Small airway damage may be present but undetectable with normal spirometry, while the patient becomes accustomed to and tolerates a persistent productive cough. However, with continued irritant exposure, this initial simple bronchitis progresses.

Secretions continue to worsen and peribronchiolar fibrosis marks the onset of obstructive bronchitis that is reflected by significant expiratory airflow limitation. At this point the patient may have tolerated years of productive cough and experienced frequent chest infections related to poor mucus clearance. COPDers are particularly susceptible to *Haemophilus influenza* and *Streptococcus pneumoniae*. The sputum is abundant and capable of plugging significant numbers of airways and may be blood tinged; COPD is the most common cause of hemoptysis. Airways may demonstrate hyperreactivity and mimic an asthmatic response.

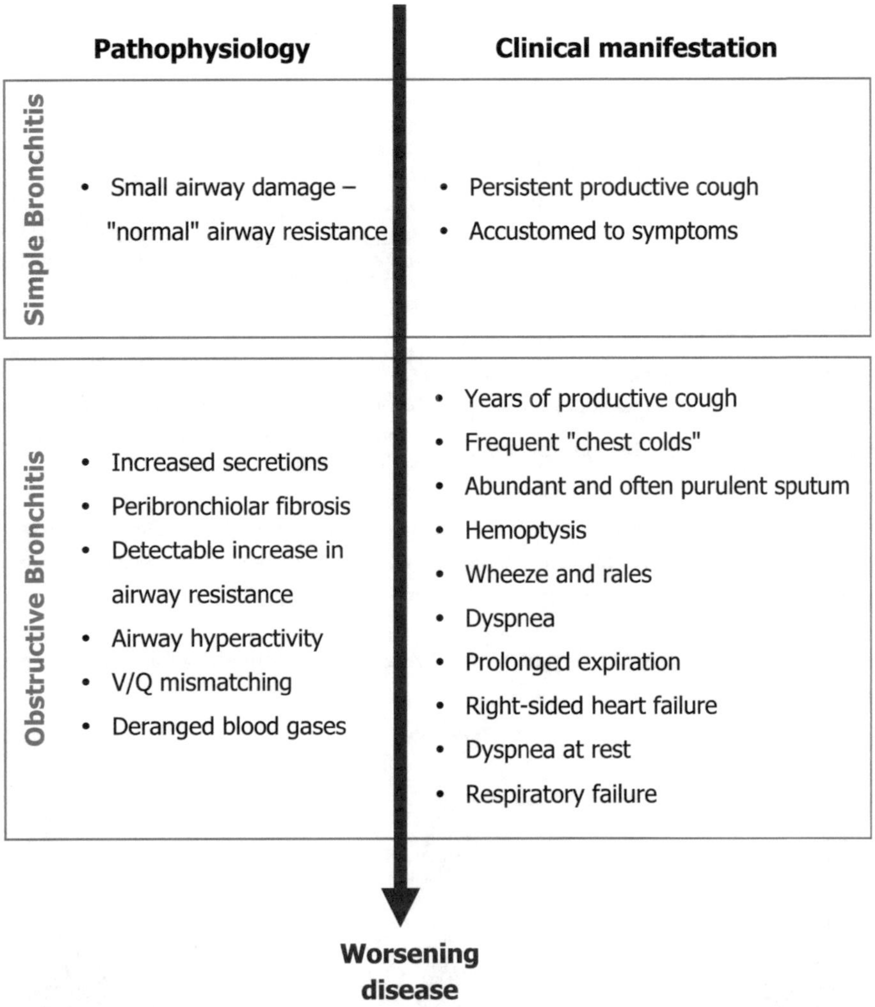

Figure 1.14: The pathophysiological and clinical events as chronic bronchitis progresses.

The onset of dyspnea is insidious and is usually first experienced during exertion—leading the patient to avoid exercise, which in turn leads to deconditioning and a worsening of the symptom. Lung sounds include **wheezes** and **rales**, the rales often clearing after cough.

With worsening airway flow limitation expiration becomes prolonged and may be incomplete due to airway collapse that leads to characteristic hyperinflation.

Mucus plugging and airway closure leads to areas of V/Q abnormalities through the lung, and localized areas of hypoxia can lead to pulmonary vasoconstriction. When significant regions of the lung are vasoconstricted, pulmonary vascular resistance can rise enough to induce right-sided heart failure.

With continued progression of the disease, blood gases become deranged as insufficient alveolar ventilation is achieved. As the disease approaches its end stage, the patient experiences dyspnea at rest until respiratory failure occurs and the patient is hypoxemic and hypercarbic.

Emphysema

Emphysema, a possible second component to COPD, involves permanent enlargement of airspaces distal to the terminal bronchioles and destruction of alveolar walls, as is evident in figure 1.15.

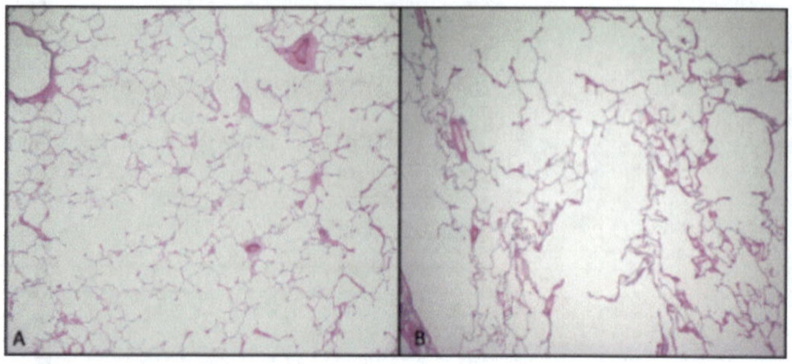

Figure 1.15: Histological comparison of normal (left) and emphysematous (right) lung tissue.

The pattern of airspace destruction varies with underlying cause and revolves around the acinus (figure 1.16), the functional unit of the lung comprised of the terminal airways and the alveoli that collectively make up the respiratory zone of the lung. In its broadest classification, emphysema can take on either a centriacinar or panacinar distribution (figure 1.16). In centriacinar emphysema, the respiratory duct is affected while the distal alveoli are mostly unaffected. This is more commonly found in the upper lung fields and associated with smoking and the concurrent presence of chronic bronchitis.

This pathology slide in figure 1.15 illustrates this pattern of tissue destruction with isolated areas of damage, surrounded by relatively normal alveolar structure.

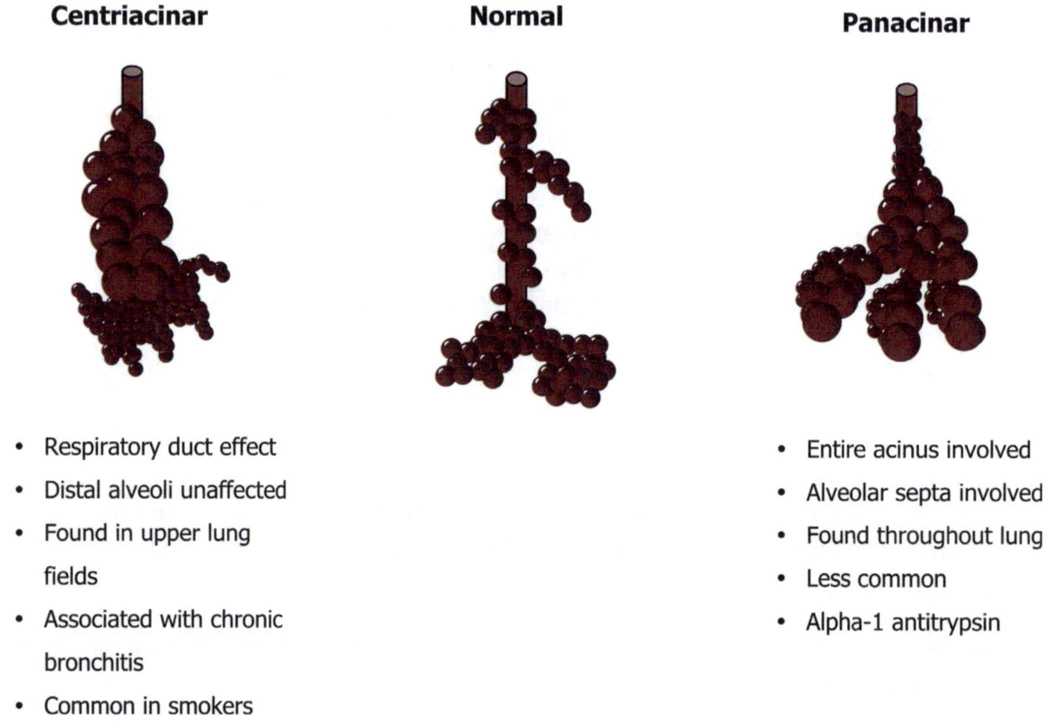

Figure 1.16: Characteristic patterns of emphysema.

Panacinar emphysema, as the name suggests, involves the entire acinus (figure 1.16), and the alveolar structure is more involved creating large airspaces that occur throughout the lung. This is evident in the pathology slide in figure 1.16 that shows much more uniform damage than the centriacinar example. Panacinar emphysema is much less common and is the pattern of destruction associated with alpha-1 antitrypsin deficiency, which we will deal with in a moment.

So having seen the morphology of emphysema, we will look at how this damage occurs.

Pathophysiology of Emphysema

The normal structure of alveoli and respiratory ducts consists of type 1 and type 2 pneumocytes with elastic fibers that contribute to the structure's mechanical behavior. Emphysema involves the loss of these parenchymal fibers.

The presence of irritants, such as cigarette smoke, causes oxidization and the dysfunction of antiprotease enzymes. Without their inhibitory action, the activity of proteases increases and causes the destruction of local tissue. One of these proteases is elastase, whose elevated activity leads to irreparable loss of parenchymal fibers.

Elastase is also released by neutrophils and macrophages that arrive in response to the inflammatory cascade caused by the inhaled smoke. This causes further destruction of elastin fibers.

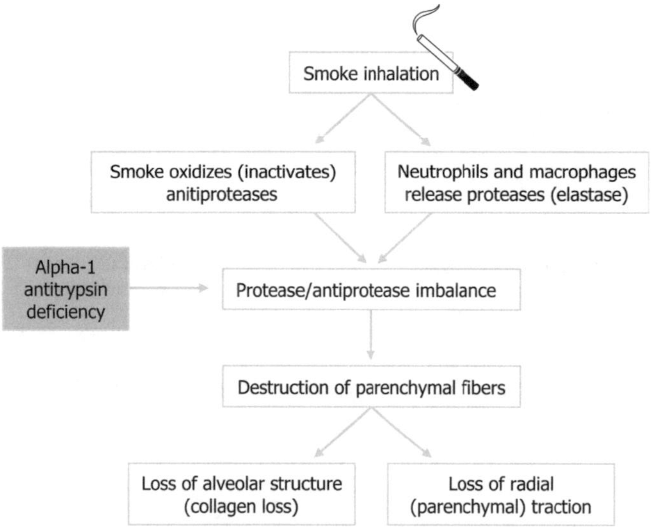

Figure 1.17: Pathological process of emphysema.

The pathogenesis of emphysema (figure 1.17) might be summarized as an imbalance between the activities of antiproteases and proteases. Antiproteases are suppressed, and proteases are elevated.

The emphysema in about 1 percent of COPD patients is caused by a genetic lack of alpha-1 anti-trypsin. Even without tobacco use, these patients have an antiprotease/protease imbalance that results in loss of elastin and collagen and produces the panacinar emphysema shown previously (figure 1.16). If an alpha1-anti-trypsin patient does smoke, this imbalance is worsened and emphysema may develop by their late twenties.

The loss of the elastic tissue and alveolar structure produces several pathophysiological changes in lung mechanics and function that result in typical clinical signs.

Clinical Presentation of Emphysema

Lung recoil is the opposing force to the chest wall's tendency to spring outward. The loss of elastin reduces lung recoil and the chest wall can move outward, producing a characteristic **"barrel-chest"** (figure 1.18).

The lack of recoil also means that passive expiration is ineffective and active expiration must be employed. The positive **pleural pressure** associated with active expiration enhances dynamic airway collapse that leads to gas trapping and characteristic **hyperinflation** (figure 1.18). To prevent this, the emphysema patient may adopt pursed lip breathing to maintain airway pressure during expiration that props open the airways.

The hyperinflation and nonuniform tissue damage can lead to a heterogenous distribution of ventilation and V/Q abnormalities that diminish gas exchange. Gas exchange will also be diminished by the enlargement of airspaces, reducing available surface area (figure 1.18).

The deterioration of gas exchange and lung mechanics worsens as more lung becomes involved, and the stage of the disease, and any concurrent chronic bronchitis, is classified by the level of airway flow limitation (e.g., FEV_1/FVC).

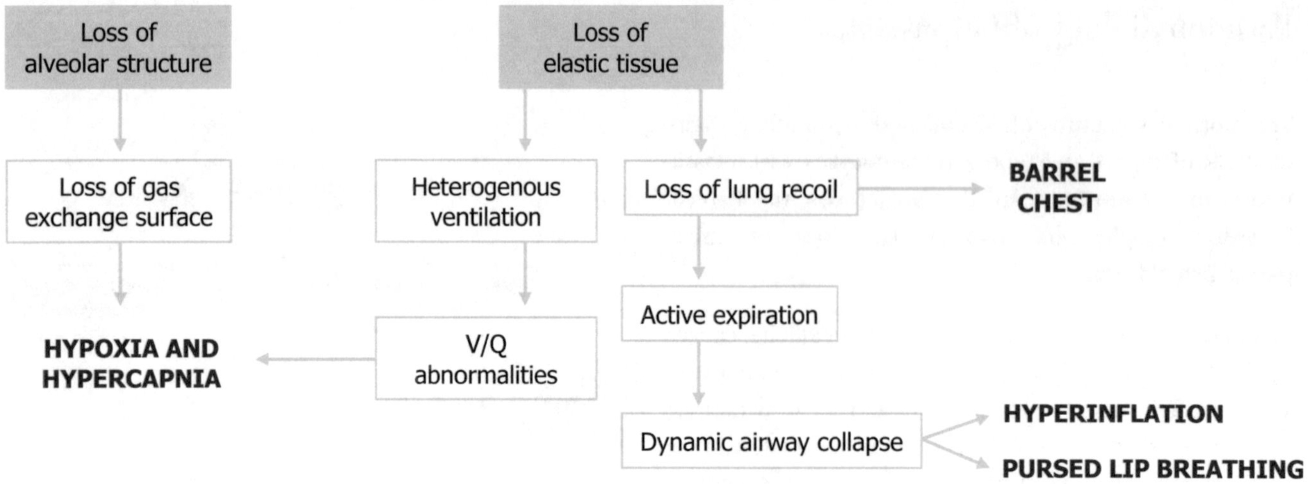

Figure 1.18: The pathophysiological events that lead to the clinical signs of emphysema.

It might also be worth noting here that COPD can produce or be associated with a number of comorbidities; we have already mentioned hypertension, but pulmonary artery disease, coronary heart disease, heart failure, lung cancer, and malnutrition may contribute to a low quality of life that is typically associated with COPD. This in turn may contribute to the high incidence of anxiety disorders and depression experienced by COPD patients.

Cystic Fibrosis

Cystic fibrosis (CF) is an inherited disorder that affects the exocrine glands of not only the lungs, but also the pancreas, intestines, and bile ducts. We will focus only on the pulmonary aspects here and see how CF produces an obstructive lung disease.

Cystic fibrosis affects the composition of the fluid lining the airways. Changes in this fluid lead to serious sequelae that dramatically shorten life expectancy. Even with modern therapy, many CF patients only live until their thirties or early forties, and some still die in infancy.

There are two hypotheses about the pathophysiological mechanism of CF: the low volume and the high salt. We will focus only on the low volume hypothesis as there is increasing evidence to support this and emerging evidence against the high salt hypothesis.

Pathophysiology of Cystic Fibrosis

Control of the airway fluid relies on the action of ion channels in the apical membranes of epithelial cells, and there are two channels to focus on: CFTR and ENaC. The CFTR channels let chloride out of the cell, while the ENaC lets sodium in (top panel, figure 1.19).

This exchange helps maintain a healthy fluid layer in the airway, but fails in CF because of a nonfunctioning CFTR channel (right panel, figure 1.19).

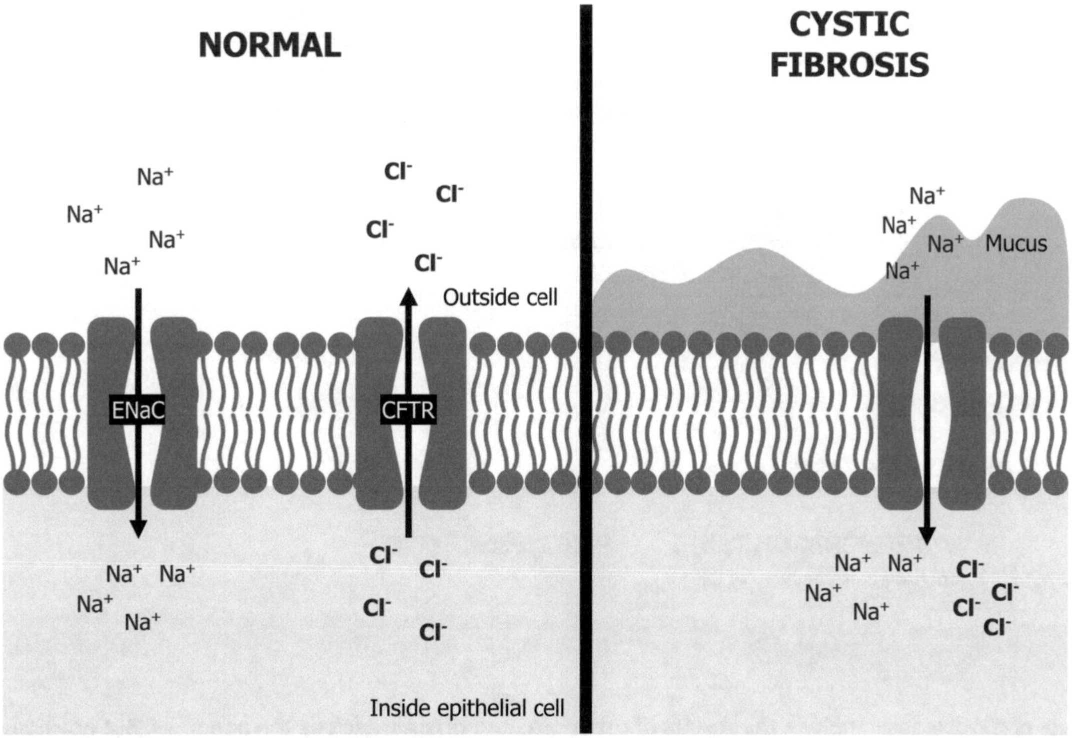

Figure 1.19: The impact of ion currents in normal and CF cells on fluid layer and cilia.

There are numerous mutations that are known to produce a dysfunctional CFTR channel, but 70 percent of CF cases are due to the delta-F-508 mutation (so named as the mutation leads to a deletion of phenylalanine at position 508 of the CFTR protein). This is a Mendelian recessive trait, and CF occurrence is 1 in 2,500 live births.

So what are the consequences of CFTR dysfunction? Chloride ends up being trapped inside the cell (bottom panel, figure 1.19), and this leads to a greater influx of sodium through the ENaC down its electrochemical gradient, leaving a higher concentration of salt inside the cells that pulls water in from the airway lumen. The low fluid volume in the airway results in:

- **viscous mucus**, and
- **collapse of cilia.**

This combination severely impacts mucus clearance (thicker, heavier mucus with compromised cillary escalator). The defective CFTR channel therefore results in mucus retention and airway obstruction. This in turn leads to reduced alveolar ventilation and repeated infections. The two most common culprits for infection in CF are *Staphylococcus aureus* and *Pseudomonsa aeruginosa.* Normal functional CFTR appears to suppress P. aeruginosa, perhaps explaining its prevalence in cystic fibrosis where it can be found in the sputum of almost all CF patients.

The consequences of repeated infection are a mixture of serious conditions and pathologies including atelectasis, pneumonia, bronchiectasis, and other structural abnormalities of the airways (figure 1.20).

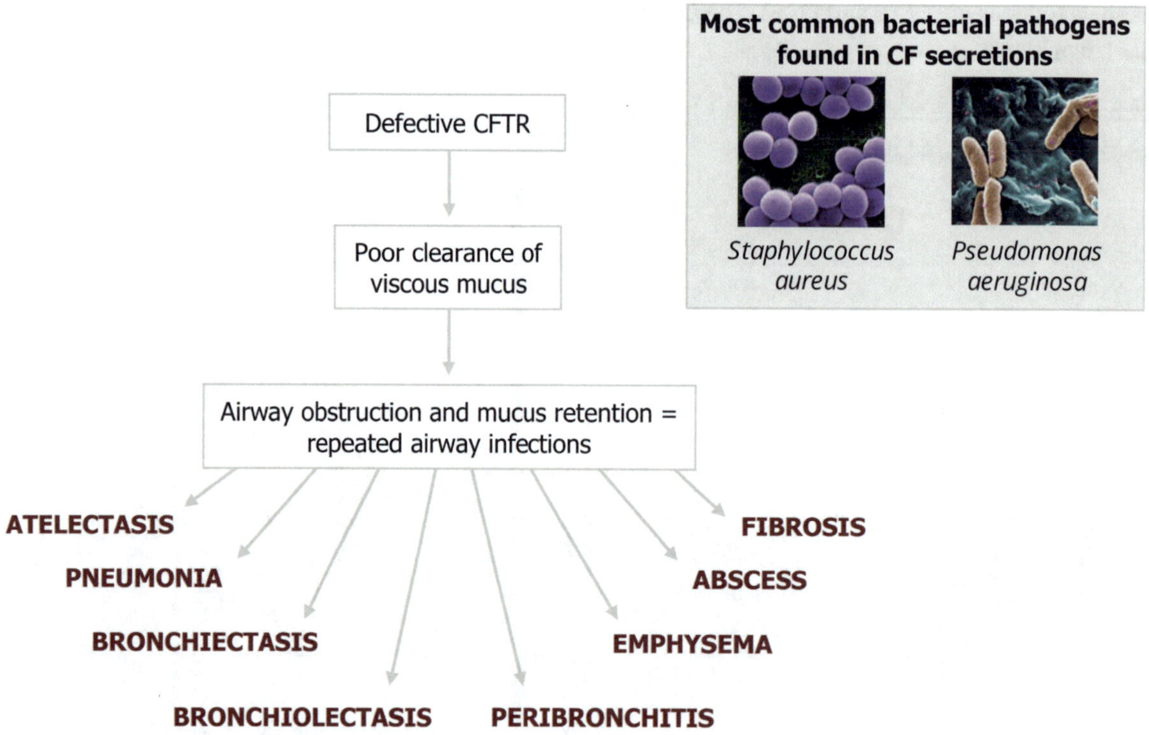

Figure 1.20: Pulmonary consequences of CF.

The findings of CF obviously include the results of other effected organs, such as the pancreas. But nowadays these are more easily addressed, and it is pulmonary involvement that still proves critical. The onset of pulmonary involvement is variable and may be weeks or years after birth.

Clinical Presentation of Cystic Fibrosis

Findings progress with progressive airway damage (figure 1.21), but start with cough that may be dry at first but transitions to productive to expel the copious, viscous mucus. With poor mucus clearance, the patient experiences repeated infections that exacerbate symptoms at each stage of the disease.

CF patients usually have an abnormal sinus x-ray and evidence of chronic sinusitis as well as a high occurrence of nasal polyps.

With increasing and irreversible airway damage, the patients begins to experience dyspnea, and the damage may lead to hemoptysis, spontaneous pneumothorax, and a barrel chested appearance. Signs of prolonged pulmonary dysfunction appear as the disease progresses, such as finger clubbing, cyanosis, and cor pulmonale (right-sided heart failure caused by lung disease). As the patient approaches respiratory failure the accessory muscles are deployed. Patients succumb to the respiratory failure or an overwhelming infection.

Because CF also affects sweat gland function, the sweat test remains a standard diagnostic with a chloride level greater than 60 mEq/L being indicative of CF. This test is more reliable in children than adults, who may have developed other conditions that affect the composition of sweat.

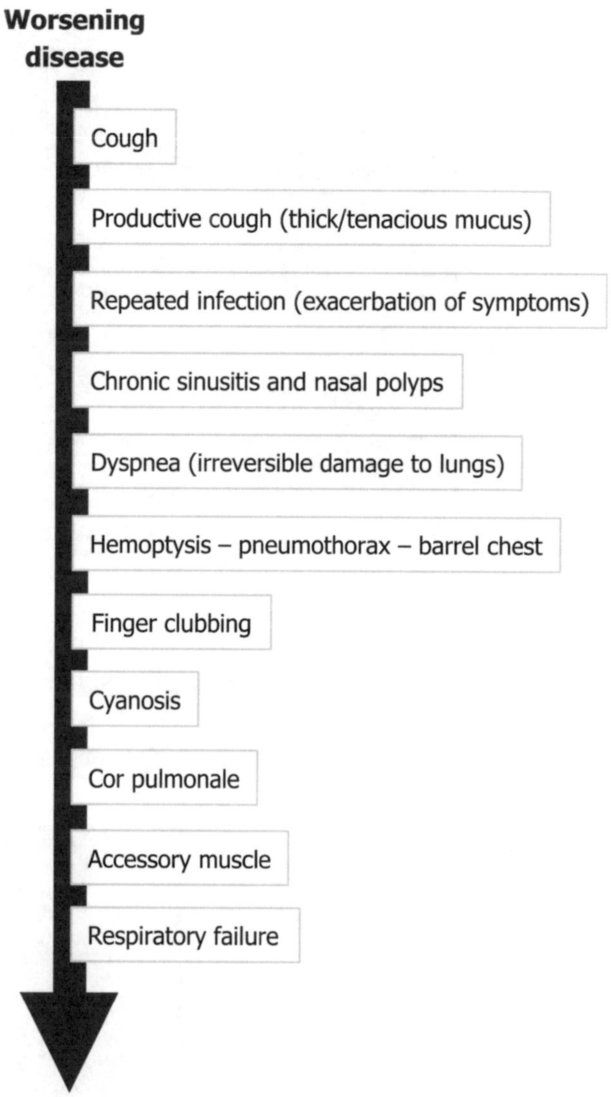

Figure 1.21: Clinical signs of the pulmonary progression of CF.

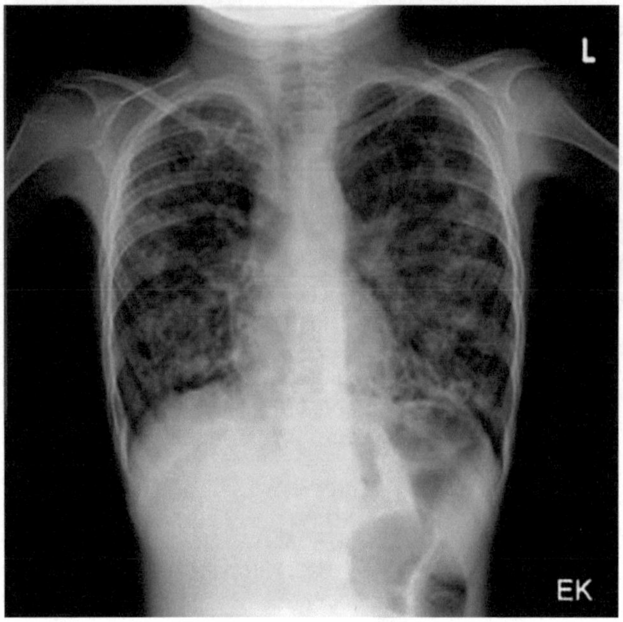

- Diffuse hyperinflation
- Increased lung markings
- Mucoid impaction
- Atelectasis
- Infiltration/abscess
- Mediastinal emphysema
- Pneumothorax

Figure 1.22: Typical chest x-ray findings of CF.

Chest x-rays show (figure 1.22) signs of hyperinflation associated with gas trapping and the hallmarks of any other complications that the CF has induced. These are viewed more clearly with the common use of high-resolution computed tomography (HRCT)(figure 1.23) to determine the type and extent of damage that may include bronchiectasis and mucus impactions.

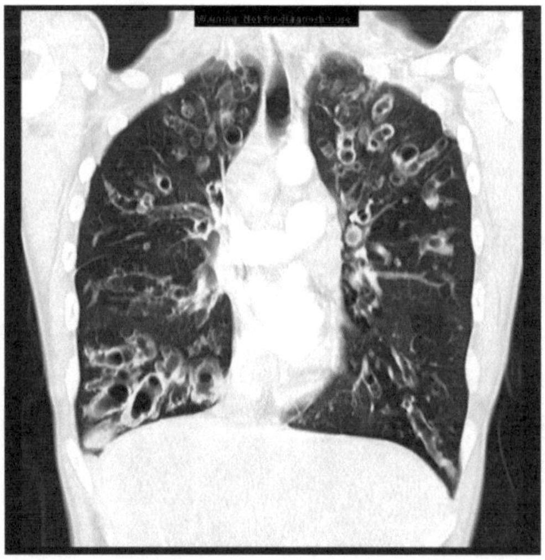

Figure 1.23: HRCT of CF lungs showing multiple, severe bronchiectasis.

Spirometry detects the airway obstruction and hyperinflation that produce a low vital capacity and high residual volume.

Bronchiectasis

This section will address bronchiectasis, a form of airway obstruction that is often a manifestation of chronic airway inflammation. Bronchiectasis involves a permanent dilation of a bronchi or bronchiole—think of bronchiectasis as the airway equivalent of an aneurysm.

A bronchiectasis starts with a section of airway wall becoming inflamed (figure 1.24), disrupting and weakening its structure. This weakening leads to a permanent dilation of the airway that impairs the clearance of secretion. Because the airway is inflamed, the amount of secretion may be significant and it begins to accumulate.

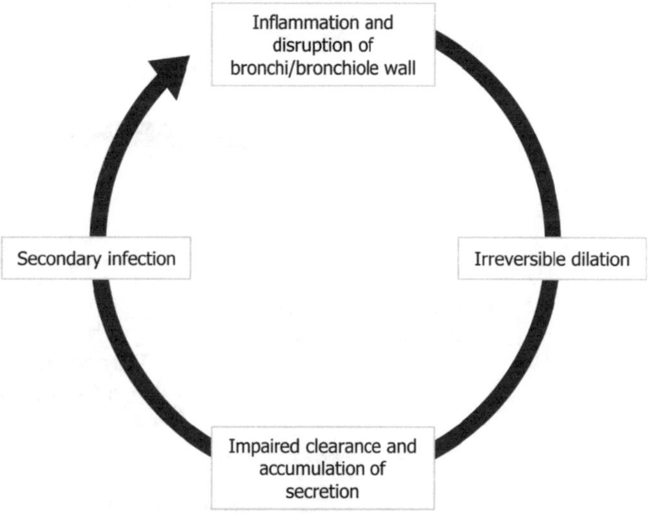

Figure 1.24: Pathophysiology of bronchiectasis.

The stagnant secretion promotes a secondary infection that leads to further inflammation, wall disruption, and dilation. Thus the airway has entered a vicious cycle that causes the dilation and retention of mucus to perpetuate (figure 1.24).

The establishing of a bronchiectasis has an initial phase leading to persistent inflammation, desquamation (which worsens the mucus clearance), and the ulceration. In what is probably a familiar story, the continued inflammation leads to fibrosis in the chronic phase of development, and this can lead to airway destruction and perhaps the condition of **bronchiolitis obliterans**.

Let us look at how this process can get started.

Pathogenesis of Bronchiectasis

There are some common culprits for initiating bronchiectasis (figure 1.25). Most start with either a decline in mucus clearance and the associated inflammation or damage to the airway wall.

About 50 percent of bronchiectasis cases are associated with cystic fibrosis where the genetic condition causes production of copious, thick mucus that is difficult to clear and often results in infection (commonly caused by *Staphylococcus aureus*).

Conditions causing cillary dyskinesia, as seen in Kartagener's syndrome, also disrupt the mucocillary escalator.

Another common cause of bronchiectasis is an allergy to *Aspergillus fumigatus*, a common fungus. In hypersensitive or immune-compromised individuals, chronic exposure can lead to allergic bronchopulmonary aspiragillosis.

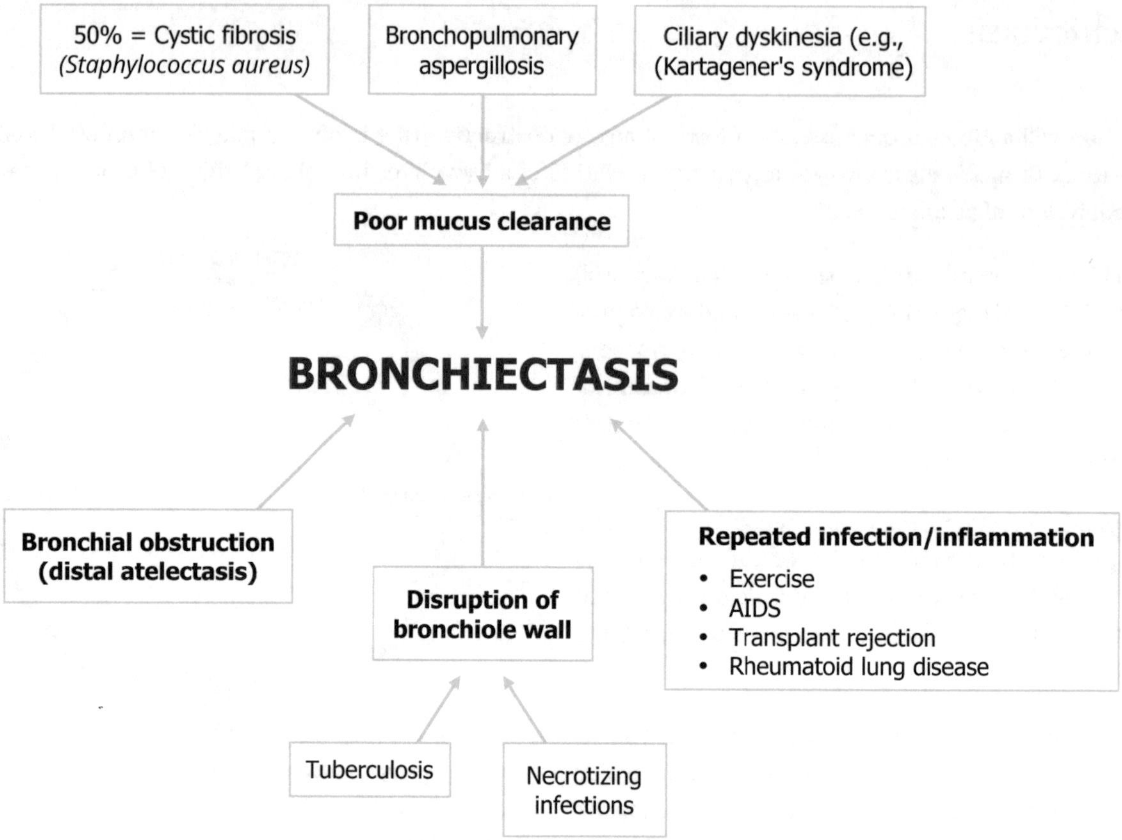

Figure 1.25: Instigating factors for bronchiectasis.

Bronchiectasis can be initiated in the vicinity of tuberculosis or other necrotizing infections that damage and weaken airway walls.

Obstruction of the bronchioles or bronchi by inhaled foreign objects, tumors, or compacted mucus can also initiate bronchiectasis through local inflammation and by preventing mucus clearance. The dilation of the airway can be worsened further by distal atelectasis that produces a negative pressure around the affected airway.

As you might have gather by now, repeated local infection or inflammation has the potential to initiate bronchiectasis, so it is perhaps not surprising that with the advent of high resolution computed tomography (CT) imaging, bronchiectasis has also been found in association with AIDS, transplant rejection, and rheumatoid lung disease.

We will now examine the results of these instigating factors.

Pathology of Bronchiectasis

The outcomes of bronchiectasis are seen in the histology slide in figure 1.26, with the affected airway lumen filled with mucus and pus, and the airway walls exhibiting fibroglandular tissue and infiltration by inflammatory cells (outer red circle).

The gross view (right panel, figure 1.26) shows severely dilated bronchi and noticeable thickening of their walls.

There are different forms of bronchiectasis; these are classified by their shape (figure 1.27).

A bronchiectasis can be cylindrical, varicose (also known as fusiform), or cystic (also known as saccular). The shape is relevant to their effect on the efficacy of coughing; cylindrical form has very little effect on cough's ability to clear mucus, whereas varicose and cystic forms tend to disproportionately collapse during cough and reduce its effectiveness at moving mucus up the airway.

As shown in figure 1.28 an x-ray shows the presence of bronchiectasis, but it can be difficult to ascertain the form. High resolution CT (figure 1.28) is better at determining the form and has all but replaced the much more invasive bronchography, which involves instillation of radiopaque medium into the tracheobronchial tree.

Where the bronchiectasis occurs in the lung is somewhat dependent on the cause. The segmental and subsegmental bronchi are the airway types most commonly affected, and the basilar segments of the lower lobes are the most frequent region in the lung. The second most common locations are the right middle lobe and lingual segments, while bronchiectasis caused by primary tuberculosis (TB) and other infections tend to occur in the upper lung fields where the infection is located (see figure 1.29).

So, how does bronchiectasis present, and what are the results of diagnostic tests?

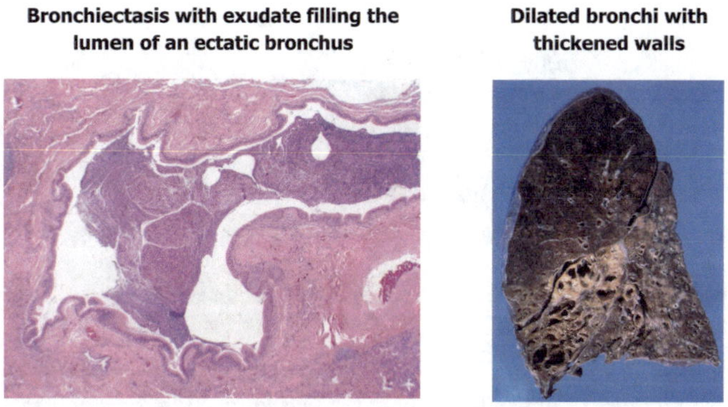

Figure 1.26: Histological and gross changes associated with severe bronchiectasis.

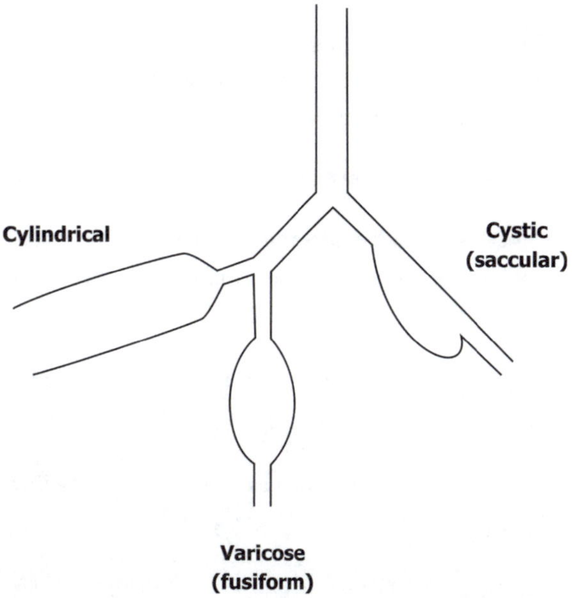

Figure 1.27: Forms of bronchiectasis.

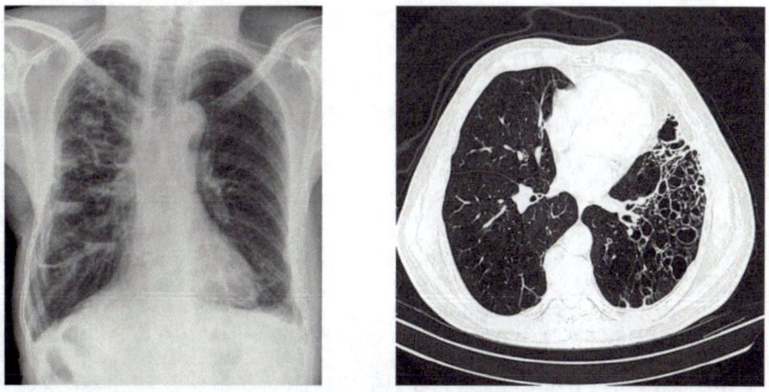

Figure 1.28: Chest x-ray and CT of severe bronchiectasis. In the x-ray there are clear markings in the right lung that follow the path of affected bronchi. The distinctly widened airways on the right of the CT are consistent with severe bronchiectasis.

Clinical Presentation of Bronchiectasis

The initial complaint is usually a persistent cough with **copious expectoration**. The amount of mucus the cough produces varies and can be as high as several hundred milliliters per day, particular when the dependent airways are involved. However, it is worth noting here that bronchiectasis in the upper lobes (usually associated with infection) may be dry with little or no mucus expectoration.

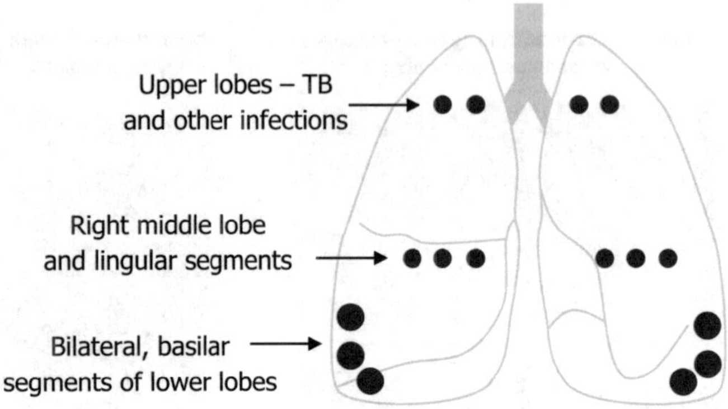

Figure 1.29: Common locations of the segmental and subsegmental broncho affected by bronchiectasis.

Generally though there is mucopurulent expectorate, and if it is associated with an anerobic infection it will likely have a foul odor. Sputum smears are loaded with white blood cells and can contain both gram-positive and -negative organisms.

The patient will likely have a history of recurrent pneumonia, the site of the pneumonia being consistent with locality of the bronchiectasis.

The expectorate may also contain blood. The degree and frequency of hemoptysis is variable and unpredictable, but occasionally it can be massive and life threatening.

The standard diagnostic tests may not be helpful in early stages, but typical signs appear with worsening airway involvement. In the early stages the patient will likely appear normal on a physical exam and have normal spirometry and arterial blood gas values. With more significant bronchiectasis, rales and rhonchi over the affected site can be heard.

Later signs with long-standing bronchiectasis include finger clubbing, but this is not exclusive to the condition.

A chest x-ray will show the peribronchial fibrosis and any atelectasis. But, as mentioned earlier, a high-resolution CT is much more effective at determining the degree and type of airway changes.

References, Resources, and Further Reading

Text

Farzan, Sattar, with Doris L. Hunsinger and Mary L. Phillips. “Chapters 8–11.” In *A Concise Handbook of Respiratory Diseases*. Reston, VA: Reston Publishing Company, 1978.

Husain, Aliya N. “Chapter 15: The Lung.” In *Robbins and Cotran Pathologic Basis of Disease*, 9th ed., edited by Vinay Kumar, Abul K. Abbas, and John C. Aster. Philadelphia: Saunders, an imprint of Elsevier Inc., 2015.

West, John B. “Chapter 4: Obstructive Diseases.” In *Pulmonary Pathophysiology: The Essentials*, 7th ed. Baltimore: Lippincott Williams & Wilkins, a Wolters Kluwer business, 2008.

Figures

Figure 1.1: Forms and prevalence of asthma. Grey, Kindred. 2022. CC BY 4.0. https://archive.org/details/1.1_20220203/mode/1up

Figure 1.2: Example of a mast cell loaded with secretory granules. Grey, Kindred. 2022. CC BY 4.0. https://archive.org/details/1.2_20220203

Figure 1.3: Vagal reflex of irritant airway receptors and the onset of asthma. Grey, Kindred. 2022. CC BY-SA 3.0. Added Mast cell by Colt browning from WikimediaCommons (CC BY-SA 3.0) and brainstem by tezar tantular from Noun Project (CC BY 3.0). https://archive.org/details/1.3_20220203

Figure 1.4: Factors promoting asthma at night. Grey, Kindred. 2022. CC BY-SA 3.0. Added FullMoon2010 by Gregory H. Revera from WikimediaCommons (CC BY-SA 3.0). https://archive.org/details/1.4_20220203

Figure 1.5: NSAIDS including aspirin shift metabolism of arachidonic acid towards bronchoconstrictive leukotrienes. Grey, Kindred. 2022. CC BY 4.0. Added see saw by Made by Made from Noun Project (CC BY 3.0). https://archive.org/details/1.5_20220203

Figure 1.6: Illustrations of normal (A), mildly asthmatic (B) and severely asthmatic (C) airways. Grey, Kindred. 2022. CC BY 4.0. https://archive.org/details/1.6_20220203

Figure 1.7: Histological signs of asthma, A = Charcot–Leyden crystals, B = Curshman's spirals. Grey, Kindred. 2022. CC BY-SA 3.0. Added Charcot-Leyden crystals, HE 2 by Patho from WikimediaCommons (CC BY-SA 3.0) and Curshman's Spiral by Doc James from WikimediaCommons (CC BY 4.0). https://archive.org/details/1.7_20220203

Figure 1.8: Components of airway remodeling in persistent asthma. Grey, Kindred. 2022. CC BY 4.0. https://archive.org/details/1.9_20220203

Figure 1.9: The progression of an asthma "attack." Grey, Kindred. 2022. CC BY 4.0. https://archive.org/details/1.8_20220203

Figure 1.10: Typical chest x-ray of asthma showing hyperlucent fields and hyperinflation. Delgado, J., Bell, D., et al. 2021. CC BY-NC-SA 3.0. "Case 1" from https://doi.org/10.53347/rID-50343.

Figure 1.11: Pathophysiology of chronic bronchitis. Grey, Kindred. 2022. CC BY 4.0. Added cigarette by Christian Frost from Noun Project (CC BY 3.0). https://archive.org/details/1.11_20220203

Figure 1.12: The Reid index compares the width of mucus glands to the width of the submucosal layer of airways. Grey, Kindred. 2022. CC BY 4.0. https://archive.org/details/1.12_20220203

Figure 1.13: Prolonged irritant exposure can lead to airway remodeling with loss of normal ciliated epithelium. Grey, Kindred. 2022. CC BY 4.0. https://archive.org/details/1.13_20220203

Figure 1.14: The pathophysiological and clinical events as chronic bronchitis progresses. Grey, Kindred. 2022. CC BY 4.0. https://archive.org/details/1.14_20220203

Figure 1.15: Histological comparison of normal (left) and emphysematous (right) lung tissue. Yuan, R., et al. "Figure 5." In "Quantification of Lung Surface Area Using Computed Tomography." *Respiratory Research* 11, no. 1 (2010): 153. Openi, CC BY 2.0.

Figure 1.16: Characteristic patterns of emphysema. Grey, Kindred. 2022. CC BY 4.0. Added Sphere by Ates Evren Aydinel from Noun Project (CC BY 3.0). https://archive.org/details/1.16_20220203

Figure 1.17: Pathological process of emphysema. Grey, Kindred. 2022. CC BY 4.0. Added cigarette by Christian Frost from Noun Project (CC BY 3.0). https://archive.org/details/1.17_20220203

Figure 1.18: The pathophysiological events that lead to the clinical signs of emphysema. Grey, Kindred. 2022. CC BY 4.0. https://archive.org/details/1.18_20220203

Figure 1.19: Ion currents in normal and CF cells impact on fluid layer and cilia. Grey, Kindred. 2022. CC BY

4.0. Added ion channel by Léa Lortal from Noun Project (CC BY 3.0). https://archive.org/details/1.19_20220203

Figure 1.20: Pulmonary consequences of CF. Grey, Kindred. 2022. CC BY 4.0. Added Staphylococcus aureus VISA 2 by Janice Haney Carr (CDC) from WikimediaCommons (public domain) and Pseudomonas by Janice Haney Carr (CDC) from WikimediaCommons (public domain). https://archive.org/details/1.20_20220203

Figure 1.21: Clinical signs of the pulmonary progression of CF. Grey, Kindred. 2022. CC BY 4.0. https://archive.org/details/1.21_20220203

Figure 1.22: Typical Chest X-ray findings of CF. Grey, Kindred. 2022. CC BY-NC-SA 3.0. Added Case 1 by Gaillard, F., Skalina, T., et al. from https://doi.org/10.53347/rID-1188 (CC BY-NC-SA 3.0). https://archive.org/details/1.22_20220203

Figure 1.23: HRCT of CF lungs showing multiple, severe bronchiectasis. Gaillard, F., El-Feky, M., et al. 2021. CC BY-NC-SA 3.0. "Case 8" from https://doi.org/10.53347/rID-8313.

Figure 1.24: Pathophysiology of bronchiectasis. Grey, Kindred. 2022. CC BY 4.0. https://archive.org/details/1.24_20220203

Figure 1.25: Instigating factors for bronchiectasis. Grey, Kindred. 2022. CC BY 4.0. https://archive.org/details/1.25_20220203

Figure 1.26: Histological and gross changes. Grey, Kindred. 2022. CC BY-SA 2.0. Added Follicular bronchiolitis associated with bronchiectasis and rheumatoid arthritis – Case 296 by Yale Rosen from Flickr (CC BY-SA 2.0) and Bronchiectasis by Yale Rosen from WikimediaCommons (CC BY-SA 2.0). https://archive.org/details/1.26_20220203

Figure 1.27: Forms of bronchiectasis. Grey, Kindred. 2022. CC BY 4.0. https://archive.org/details/1.27_20220203

Figure 1.28: Chest x-ray and computed tomography of severe bronchiectasis. Bickle, I., Niknejad, M., et al. T. 2021. CC BY-NC-SA 3.0. "Case 1" and "Case 3" from https://doi.org/10.53347/rID-50703.

Figure 1.29: Common locations of the segmental and sub-segmental broncho affected by bronchiectasis. Grey, Kindred. 2022. CC BY 4.0. https://archive.org/details/1.29_20220203

2. Upper Airway Infections

Learning objectives

- List the common viral and bacterial agents associated with upper airway infections.
- Describe the pathological events associated with an upper airway infection and how it may progress into other regions of the respiratory tract.

While the most prevalent upper respiratory tract infection (URI) is the self-limited "common cold," other less frequently occurring forms can have more serious consequences. Differentiating between the "common cold" and more consequential infections is therefore a clinical goal.

First, a quick reminder of the region we are talking about. The upper airway encompasses the extrathoracic respiratory tract, so includes the nasal cavity, paranasal sinuses, pharynx, and sometimes the larynx (figure 2.1). The lower airway starts from the trachea and includes all downstream structures.

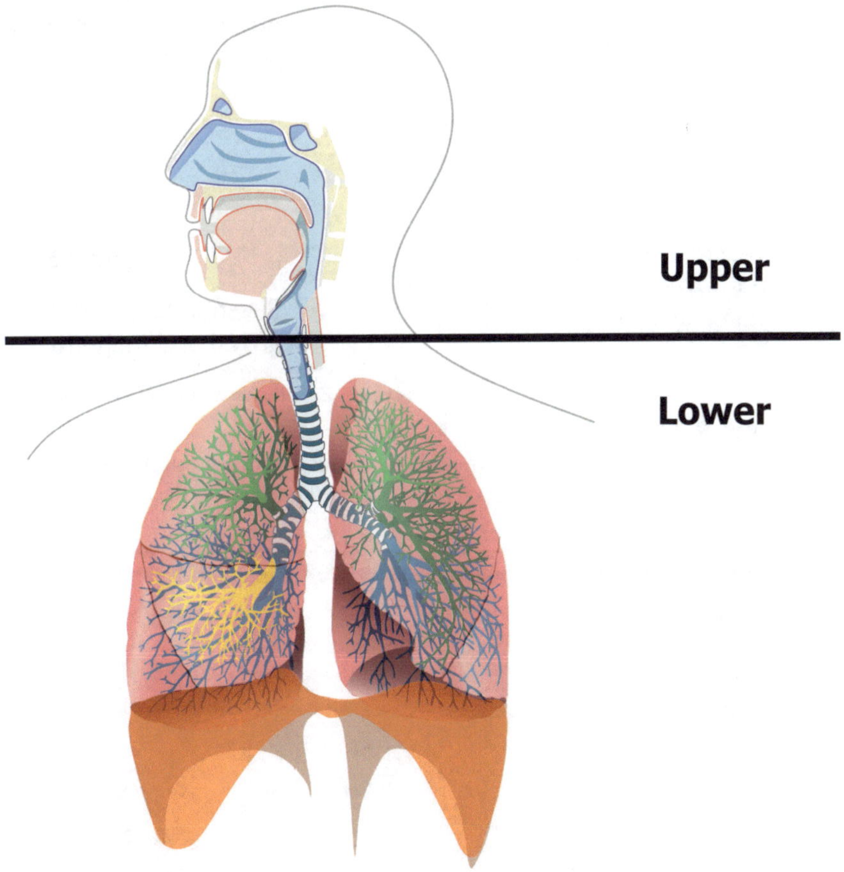

Figure 2.1: The upper airway encompasses the respiratory tract above the trachea.

The Common Cold

As with most URIs the common cold is caused by a viral infection, and although there are several different viral candidates for causing a common cold, the pathophysiological mechanism and symptoms are the same regardless of the type. This is because it is the **innate immune response**, rather than the direct infection, that is responsible for most of the symptoms.

Looking at the sequence of events involved in "getting a cold" (figure 2.2), we start with delivery of the pathogen to the upper airway and inoculation. The most common modes of delivery are hand-to-nose or hand-to-mouth contact or inhalation of aerosolized nasal fluid produced from a sneeze of an infected person. The causal virus is rarely found in saliva, so infection is spread from snot not spit.

Once in the upper airway, and if the pathogen can breach the innate defenses here (mucus and the mucociliary escalator), the virus attaches to, and then enters, the epithelial cells. In response, the invaded epithelial cells release cytokines to instigate an immune response. The primary cytokine released in this scenario is IL-8, which causes the attraction and accumulation of polymorphonuclear cells (PMN).

It is the substantial increase in PMN cells that is responsible for most of the symptoms of a common cold—runny nose, postnasal drip, and other signs of epithelial inflammation.

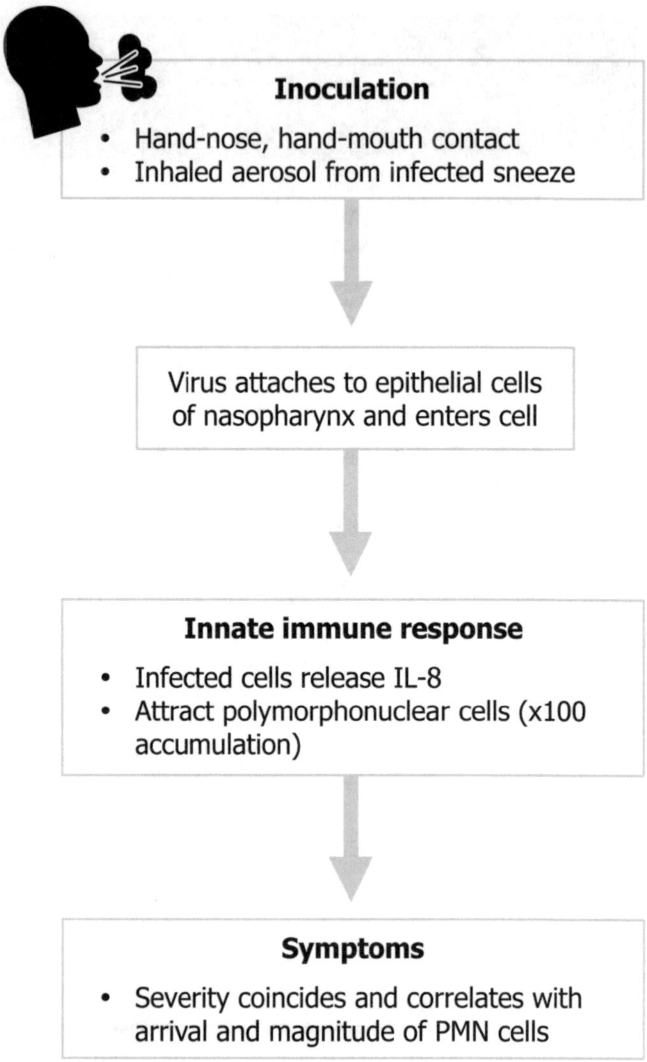

Figure 2.2: Pathophysiology of the common cold.

By far the most common cause of the common cold is the rhinovirus, followed by coronavirus and influenza, then less frequently by parainfluenza respiratory syncytial virus (RSV), and then rarely by adenovirus or enterovirus (table 2.1).

Virus	Estimated proportion in common cold	Spring	Summer	Fall	Winter
Rhinovirus	30-50%	Yes		Yes	
Coronavirus	10-15%				Yes
Influenza	5-15%	Yes			Yes
Parainfluenza	5%	Yes			
Respiratory syncytial virus	5%	Yes			Yes
Adenovirus	5%	Yes	Yes	Yes	Yes
Enterovirus	5%		Yes	Yes	

Table 2.1: The viral pathogens.

Seasonal differences (table 2.1) in the prevalence of these pathogens might help you identify the causal agent, but as the viral infections are self-limiting it is more important to ensure there is no bacterial involvement.

A viral infection can progress and cause more specific conditions than a cold, and these are identified by their location.

Rhinosinusitis

Rhinosinusitis is most commonly caused by a viral infection, and despite popular belief is only rarely associated with a concurrent bacterial infection in adults. The lining of the nasal and sinus cavities becomes inflamed, again as a result of the immune response rather than a direct effect of the virus. The congestion can be painful, but symptoms can be treated with over-the-counter analgesics. Like the common cold, the condition is self-limiting and normally resolves in seven to ten days.

Pharyngitis

When the pharynx is involved the local inflammation will cause the patient to present with a sore throat and a hoarse voice. Pharyngitis is most commonly caused by viral infection, but more serious bacterial infections (e.g., *Streptococcus*) should be considered. The two infection types are easily distinguished with tonsillar exudate and petechial mottling of the soft palate being present in a bacterial infection, but absent in a viral infection. Treatment of viral pharyngitis is limited to symptom relief, and antibiotics should be avoided.

Viral Croup

Involvement of the larynx and subglottic airway will produce croup. There are numerous causes of croup and subclassifications depending on the region involved. Viral croup, like other forms, involves inflammation of the larynx that causes the airway to narrow. Edematous airway walls form an upper airway obstruction that produces stridor. **Stridor** is a crow-like airway sound, and the phase of breathing that it appears in can be helpful in determining the site of obstruction. Stridor during inspiration is indicative of airway collapse above the vocal cords (i.e., extrathoracic), and expiratory stridor suggests a tracheal or bronchial obstruction (i.e., intrathoracic). The constriction of the airway can be seen on x-ray when severe and the narrowing produces a characteristic "steeple" sign in the trachea (see figure 2.3).

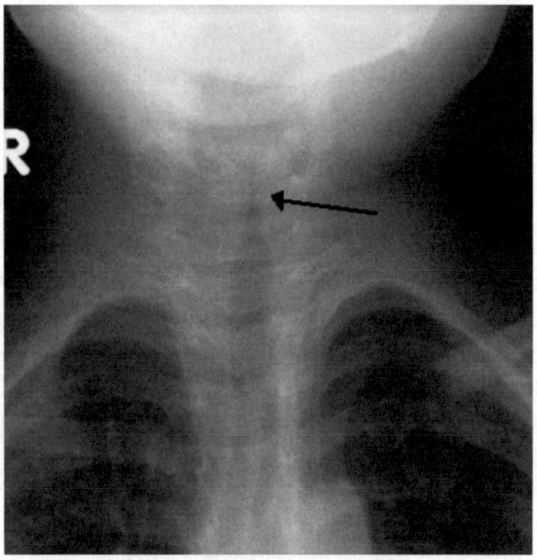

Figure 2.3: An x-ray of the upper airway of a child suffering from tracheal croup. The arrow points to a narrowing of the trachea that produces a characteristic "steeple" sign as the constriction looks like the pointed steeple of a church building.

Bacterial Infection of the Upper Airway

The induction of upper airway infection by bacteria is similar to that by virus with droplet inhalation or hand-to-mouth or nose contact. Cell adherence is usually promoted by bacterial properties, but it is bacterial toxins that instigate the signs and symptoms of infection rather than the innate immune system. We will now cover four bacteria that are capable of causing an upper airway infection.

Group A *Streptococcus*

The pathogenic mechanisms of Group A *Streptococcus* are poorly understood—partly because of the numerous and complex ways it interacts with its human host. Its coat protects it from phagocytosis, antibody binding, and opsonization. It is capable of releasing a cocktail of cell-lysing toxins as well as pyrogenic exotoxins that:

- induce lymphocyte production,
- suppress antibody synthesis, and
- induce fever.

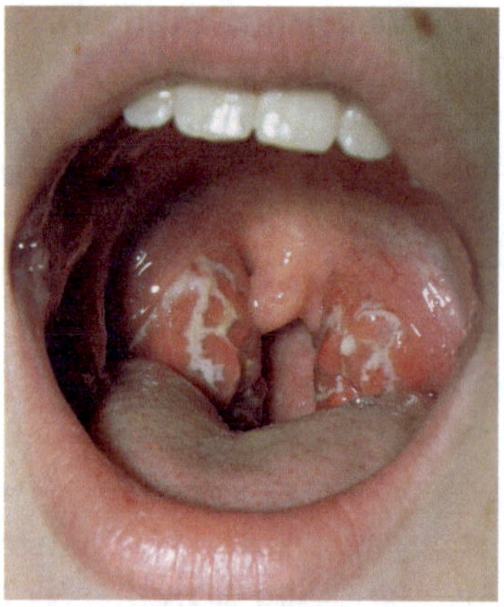

Figure 2.4: Typical signs of "strep throat."

In terms of the upper airway it is the leading cause of tonsillopharyngitis in both adults and children. A sore throat may be accompanied by fever, headache, and vomiting. Inflamed tonsils and uvula may be coated in exudates, and palatal petechiae (figure 2.4) may be be present as well as a scarlatiniform rash. Symptoms resolve in three to five days, but antibiotic therapy should be used to reduce the risk of complications that include peritonsillar cellulitis, otitis media, sinusitis, and even acute rheumatic fever.

Corynebacterium diphtheriae

After inoculation, *C. diphtheriae* releases diphtheria exotoxin and enters the cell by exploiting a membrane receptor. Once inside, the exotoxin inactivates elongation factor 2, halting protein production and causing cell death. Occurrence of diphtheria is now rare in developed countries because of vaccination programs, but infection produces sore throat, swelling of cervical lymph glands, and low-grade fever. Most cases are tonsillopharyngeal where a pseudomembrane and exudate (figure 2.5) is produced that can spread to other areas. In severe cases the spread can lead to the bull neck of diphtheria (figure 2.5) as swelling and pseudomembranes accumulate and swallowing can become difficult. If the infection becomes systemic, cardiac, neural, and renal issues may arise, including myocarditis, local neuropathies, and in severe cases renal failure.

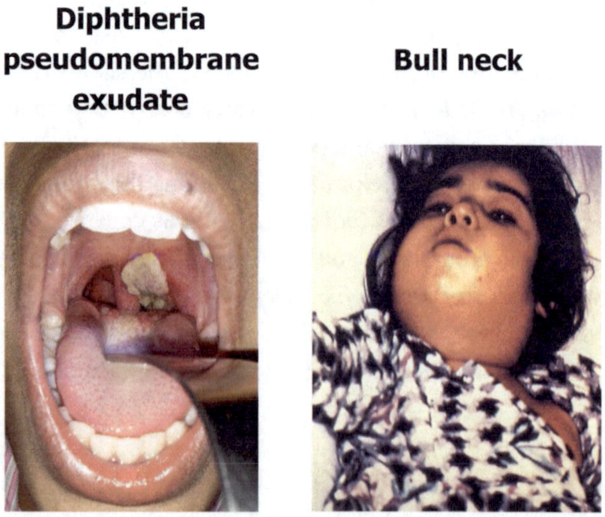

Figure 2.5: Clinical signs of C. diphtheriae: pseudomembrane exudate (left) and bull neck (right).

Bordetella pertussis

After inhalation, *B. pertussis* attaches to airway cells through a variety of adhesion molecules. The organism then releases cytotoxins that cause loss of protective respiratory cells and promote microaspiration and a distinct and prolonged cough. Pertussis's nickname of whooping cough comes from the distinct inspiratory noise. The paroxysmal stage of pertussis (that involving cough) can last between two and ten weeks, and this prolongation is likely due to the bacteria penetrating deeper regions of the lung (the cytotoxins have been found in alveolar macrophages). The disease can be life threatening to infants, but widespread vaccinations started in the forties dramatically reduced its incidence.

Haemophilus influenzae

The outer coat of the *H. influenzae* contains several proteins that attach to upper airway cells and specifically promote pharyngeal and the middle ear colonization. The outer coat also acts as an endotoxin and elicits a potent inflammatory response to produce the symptoms of the infection. Prior to routine vaccination, vascular invasion by the pathogen could produce metastatic foci including meningitis, septic arthritis, osteomyelitis, and cellulitis. Today, while upper airway infection can lead to pneumonia, the incidence of bacteremia is low.

References, Resources, and Further Reading

Text

Thomas, Micah, and Paul A. Bomar. *Upper Respiratory Tract Infection.* Treasure Island, FL: StatPearls Publishing, 2022. https://www.ncbi.nlm.nih.gov/books/NBK532961, CC BY 4.0.

Figures

Figure 2.1: The upper airway encompasses the respiratory tract above the trachea. Grey, Kindred. 2022. CC BY 4.0. Includes Respiratory system complete en by LadyofHats from WikimediaCommons (public domain). https://archive.org/details/2.1_20220203

Figure 2.2: Pathophysiology of the common cold. Grey, Kindred. 2022. CC BY 4.0. Added flu by Vectorstall from Noun Project (CC BY 3.0). https://archive.org/details/2.2_20220203

Figure 2.3: An x-ray of the upper airway of a child suffering from tracheal croup. Gaillard, Frank. 2010. CC BY-SA 3.0. "Croup Steeple Sign" from WikimediaCommons.

Figure 2.4: Typical signs of "strep throat." Heilman, James. 2010. CC BY-SA 3.0. "Pos Strep" from WikimediaCommons.

Figure 2.5: Clinical signs of c. diphtheriae: pseudomembrane exudate (upper), and bull-neck (lower). Grey, Kindred. 2022. CC BY-SA 3.0. Added Dirty white pseudomembrane classically seen in diphtheria 2013-07-06 11-07 by Dileepunnikri from WikimediaCommons (CC BY-SA 3.0) and Diphtheria bull neck.5325 lores by CDC from WikimediaCommons (public domain). https://archive.org/details/2.5_20220203

3. Lower Airway Infections

Learning objectives

- Describe three types of lower airway infection and their pathophysiology.
- Categorize pneumonia on a histological, anatomical, and etiological basis.
- List the clinical findings associated with pneumonia.

Despite being open to the external environment, lower airway infections are relatively rare because of the lungs, multitiered defense systems. However, these defenses can be breached if they are weakened or the presentation of a pathogen is overwhelming.

The site of the infection in the lower airways determines the form and severity of the disease. Infection of the trachea and bronchi produces **acute bronchitis**. Deeper into the airways and the infection produces acute **infectious bronchiolitis**, and deeper still, when infection reaches the air ducts and alveoli, we have **pneumonia**. Because pneumonia involves the gas exchange surfaces these infections tend to be most severe, and consequently we will spend most of this chapter on them. But first we will look at acute bronchitis and acute infectious bronchiolitis.

Acute Bronchitis

Acute bronchitis often originates from a migrating upper airway infection, and hence the usual candidates for a URI are the pathogens associated with acute bronchitis, and most are viral but can include mycoplasma infection. Acute bronchitis can be caused by bacteria, but it is usually an opportunistic secondary infection by resident bacteria taking advantage of a weakened airway. Regardless of the pathogen, let us look at the sequence of pathophysiological events in acute bronchitis (figure 3.1).

First the bronchial mucus membranes become inflamed. Taking a careful history can help you distinguish infectious causes from other instigators of airway inflammation, such as physical or chemical insults or an allergic response. The inflammation will initially produce a dry cough, but within two to three days bronchial secretions will be established, the cough will become productive, and rales can be heard over the site of the infection, which constitutes the clinical diagnosis.

The inflamed airways may also become hyperreactive, and this may compound any concurrent allergic response or existing asthma resulting in **bronchospasm** and **wheeze**. See figure 3.1 for a summary.

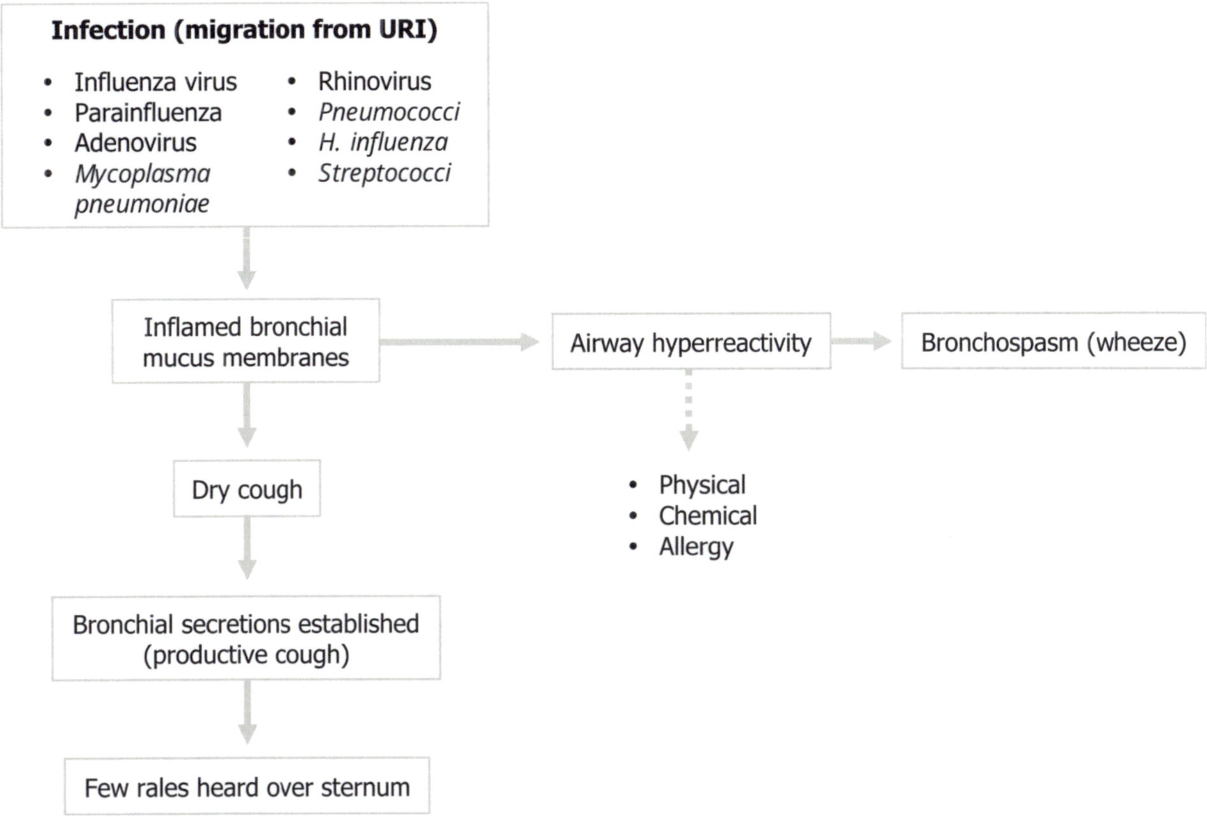

Figure 3.1: Pathophysiology of acute bronchitis.

Infectious Bronchiolitis

Penetrating deeper into the airway a pathogen can cause acute infectious bronchiolitis. By far the most common culprit is **respiratory syncytial virus (RSV)**. This is the most common cause of lower airway infection in children under one year old and is estimated to cause more infant deaths than any other pathogen with the exception of malaria. While it can affect adults, it usually occurs only in the elderly and immunosuppressed patients.

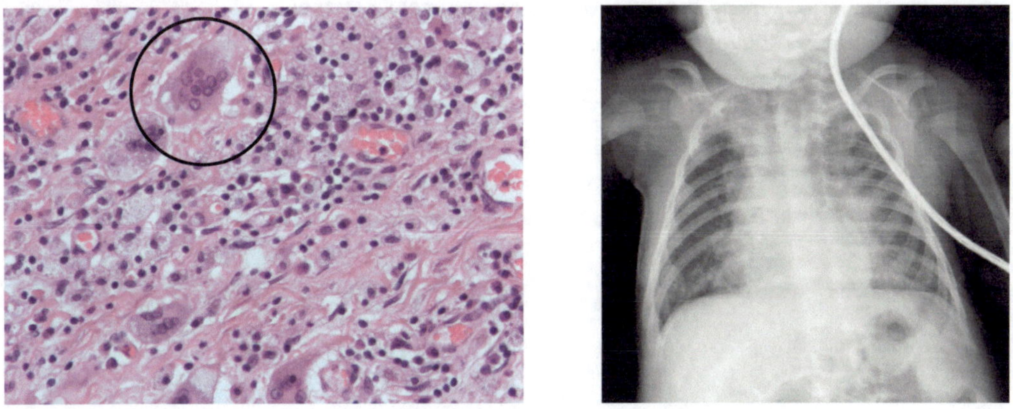

Figure 3.2: Histological and radiographic findings for an RSV infection. The left panel shows syncytial giant cells (circled). The right panel shows an x-ray of a child with RSV where densities folow bronchi and a flattened diaphragm.

Infection starts in the nasopharynx and then progresses to the epithelium of the bronchioles that appears particularly susceptible to RSV infection. Immune cells are called to the area, but the predominant feature of the infection is the sloughing of the bronchiolar epithelium and the appearance of **syncytial giant cells** in the airway lumen, as seen in the insert of the histology slide in figure 3.2. With anatomically smaller bronchioles, infants are susceptible to this epithelial sludge blocking the airway. The hallmark of the infection reflects the obstructive nature of the disease with hyperinflation.

The young patient will likely present with a recent history of cough and hallmarks of shortness of breath such as use of accessory muscles. A scattered wheeze is likely, and in severe cases the child develops an **expiratory grunt**.

Unresolved the RSV can spread to type 1 and 2 pneumocytes through cell-to-cell transmission. There is a high incidence of apnea associated with RSV infection, presumably due to the virus activating defensive reflexes associated with the larynx.

Pneumonia

Now we will look at the consequences of infection of the terminal airways and what is referred to as pneumonia. Although pneumonia can result from infection by one of any number of pathogens, we will first look at a generalized pathophysiological mechanism.

The pathogen arrives in the alveolar space causing activation of alveolar macrophages and recruitment of neutrophils from the bloodstream. These first responder cells release cytokines to attract more neutrophils and hyperpermeabilize the vasculature. Consequently the airspace becomes congested with pathogens, neutrophils, and exudate and incapable of being ventilated (figure 3.3). This produces **V/Q mismatching** in the effected area and the potential for the establishing of **intrapulmonary shunts**.

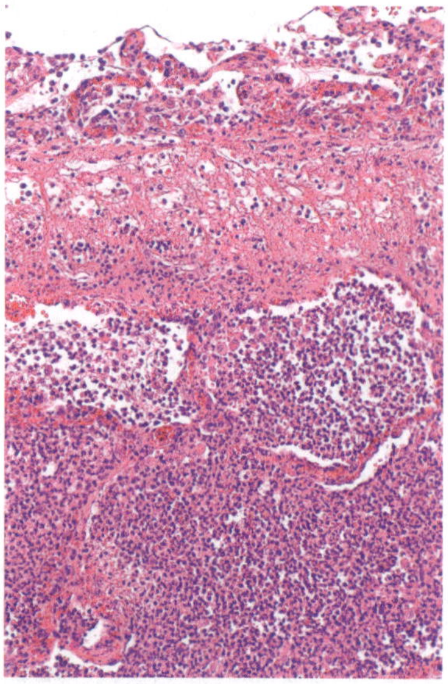

Figure 3.3: Neutrophils, bacteria, and exudate occupy airspaces in a typical pneumonia.

The infection may not be retained by the airway structure and can penetrate the pleural space, in which case an effusion is likely.

The pneumonia-causing pathogen can often be found in blood analysis but the patient remains asymptomatic, but if the infection becomes more established significant signs and symptoms of bacteremia arise.

An infection may lead to necrotized tissue and formation of an abscess in the lung. The prevalence of this is mostly dependent on the pathogen; for example, a tuberculosis infection is famous for causing walled-off abscesses (or granuloma) that try to contain the mycobacterium. These processes are summarized in figure 3.4.

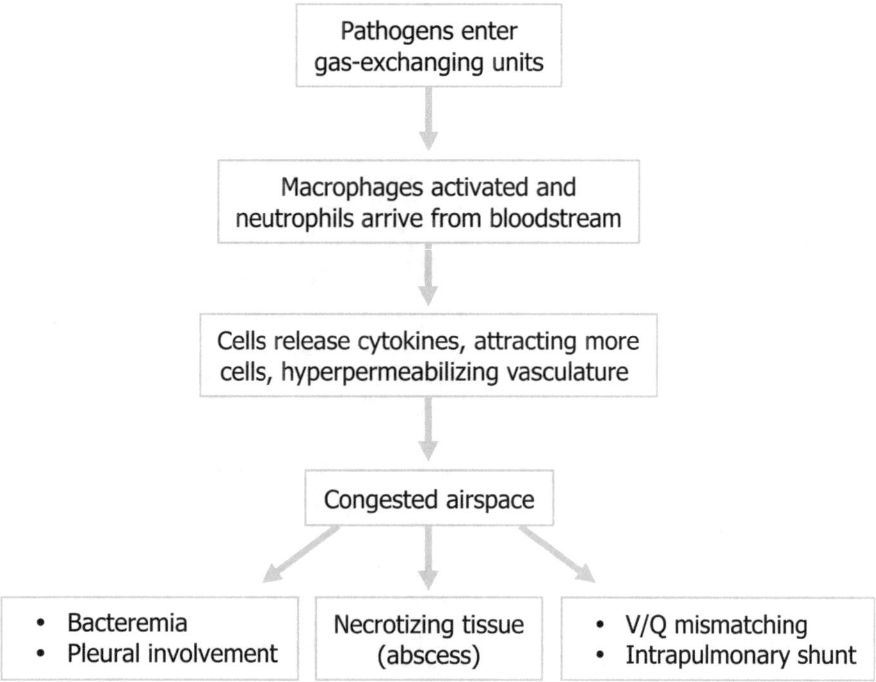

Figure 3.4: General pathophysiology of pneumonia.

Classification of Pneumonia

The causes of pneumonia are many, but so are the ways in which they are classified. Pneumonias are distinguished by:

- where the patient became infected,
- where in the lung the infection is established, and
- where the pathogen resides at a cellular level.

Typical or atypical pneumonia: We can start at arguably the *least* clinically helpful classification, the microscopic location. Pneumonias can be either **typical** or **atypical**. Typical pneumonium involves the presence of pathogens and immune cells in the airspace, whereas atypical has the pathogen and inflammatory response within the alveolar walls and interstitium (table 3.1). The site is usually dictated by the mode of the pathogen, with typical pneumonia being bacterial and atypical being caused by virus or mycobacterium that are capable of entering cells.

The two forms can have different signs and symptoms with typical pneumonia having a more rapid onset and atypical being more gradual. Both can be associated with fever, but extrapulmonary features such as headache, joint and muscle pain, and nausea are more characteristic of atypical pneumonia. Because of the location of the pathogen; typical pneumonia is associated with a productive cough, whereas the cough of atypical pneumonia is dry, as summarized in table 3.1.

On x-ray the atypical pneumonia shows more diffuse patchy markings associated with the infiltrated interstitium, whereas an x-ray of typical pneumonia shows lobar opacities caused by consolidated airspaces (table 3.1).

Typical pneumonia	Atypical pneumonia
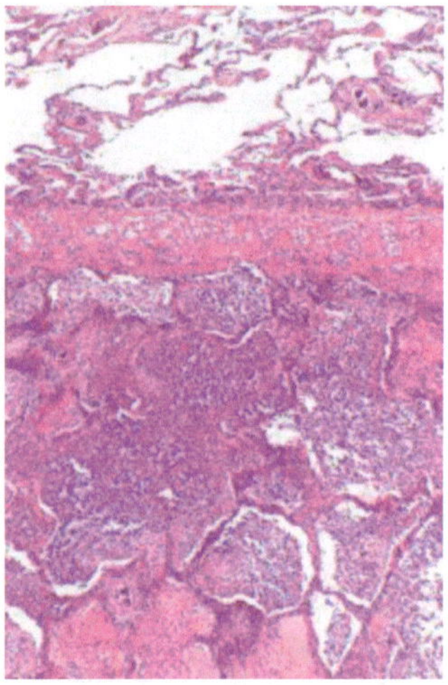	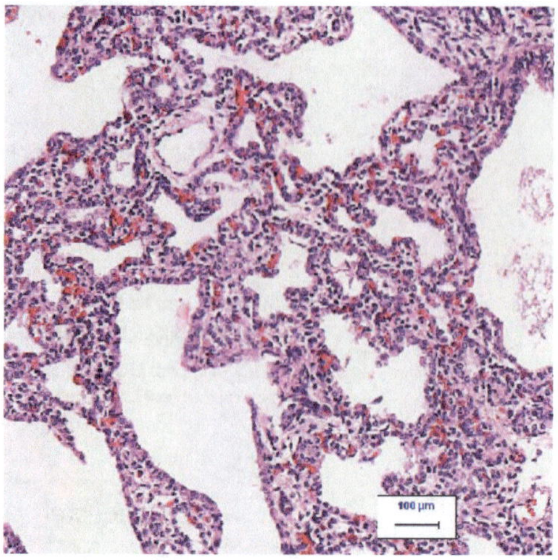
- Airspace involvement - Bacterial - Rapid onset - Few extrapulmonary features - Productive cough	- Interstitial involvement - Viral/mycoplasma - Gradual onset - Extra-pulmonary features - Dry cough
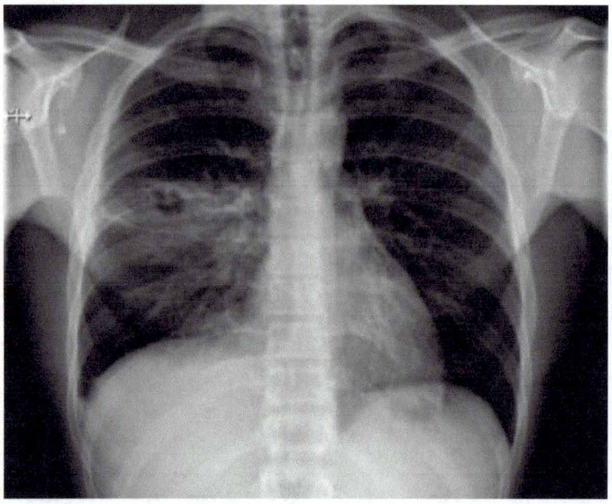	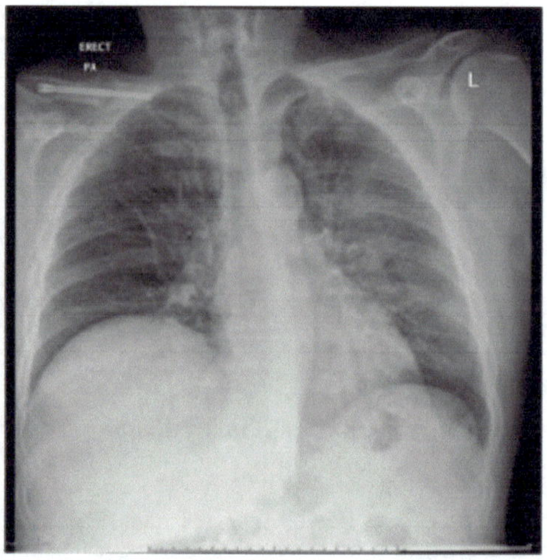

Table 3.1: Comparison of typical and atypical pneumonia.

Bronchopneumonia or lobar pneumonia: The next classification is based on the infection's gross location—whether it occurs in a bronchiolocentric pattern to produce **bronchopneumonia**, or whether the consolidation occurs in continuous airspaces to occupy a lobe to produce **lobar pneumonia**. Bronchopneumonia will produce distinct areas of infiltrate, and the chest x-ray will reflect this with opacities following the effected airways (table 3.2). Lobar pneumonia will involve dense consolidation outlining the whole lobe and the possibility of air brochograms as air-filled bronchi are surrounded by the infiltrated, more dense alveoli (table 3.2). Bronchopneumonia is usually bilateral, whereas lobar pneumonia tends to be unilateral. However, both can exist in the same patient, as is the case in the example x-ray in table 3.2.

Bronchopneumonia	Lobar pneumonia
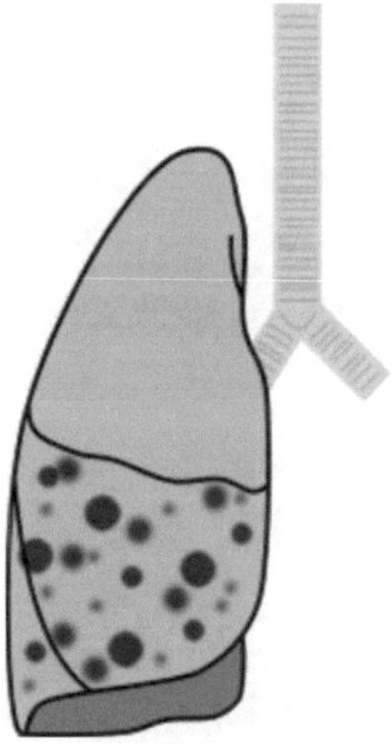	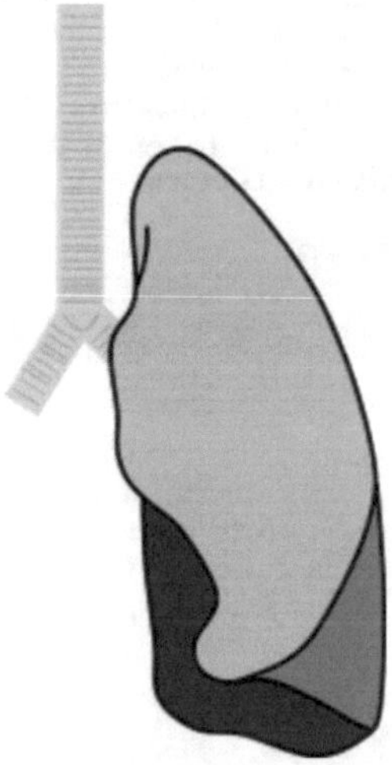
- Multiple distinct foci around bronchioles - Usually bilateral	- Dense consolidation (air bronchograms) - Usually unilateral
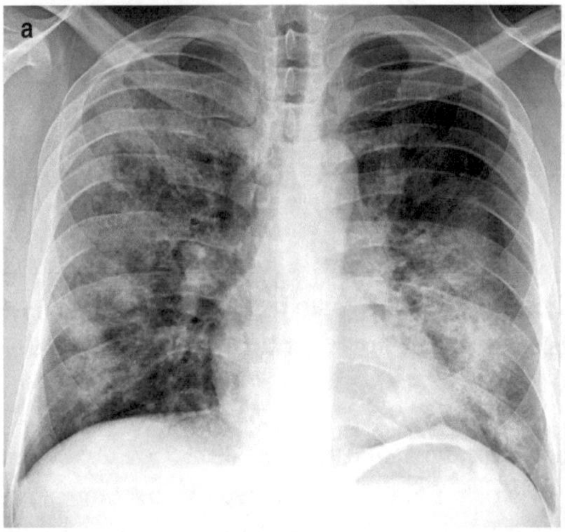	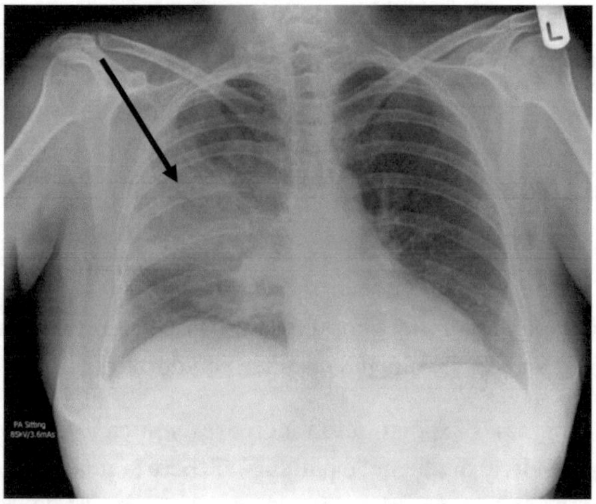

Table 3.2: Comparison of bronchopneumonia and lobar pneumonia.

Hospital-acquired or community-acquired pneumonia: The last classification relates to the setting in which the infection was acquired, either out in the community or during hospitalization. This classification can provide clues to identifying the pathogen involved. By far the most common cause of community-acquired pneumonia is *Streptococcus pneumoniae*. Other pathogens can be responsible but tend to affect only those with an underlying condition or characteristic; they are listed in table 3.3 with the usual instigating issue in parentheses. Legionella-related pneumonia requires exposure to laced water droplets, and mycoplasma infection tends to affect young adults living in close quarters, such as military barracks or college dorms. Lastly, and more uncommonly, the pneumonia may be caused by a viral infection.

Hospital-acquired pneumonia is defined as occurring at least three days after hospitalization. Unlike community-acquired pneumonias the pathogen is frequently a gram-negative bacteria or staphylococci that normally would not be able to become established in the lung. However, the hospitalized patient's weakened state of health, state of consciousness, exposure to poor sterile technique for intubation, or antibiotic therapy can provide these listed pathogens an opportunity (table 3.3).

Community-acquired	**Hospital-acquired** **- Contracted >3 days of hospitalization** **- Gram-negative bacteria and staphylococci** **- Patient is in poor health** **- Poor state of consciousness (aspiration)** **- Defective defense mechanisms** **- Poor antibiotic therapy**
Streptococcus pneumoniae	*Escherichia coli*
Haemophilus influenzae (COPD)	*Enterobacter*
Moraxella catarrhalis (COPD)	*Proteus*
Klebsiella pneumoniae (alcoholics)	*Serratia*
Staphylococcus (infants, IV drug abuse)	*Haemophilus influenzae*
Escherichia coli (alcoholics, diabetics)	*Pseudomonas*
Legionella pneumophila (water droplets)	*Acinetobacter*
Mycoplasma pneumoniae (young adults)	*Staphylococcus*
Influenza, varicella zoster, adenovirus	*Streptococcus pneumoniae*
	Klebsiella pneumoniae

Table 3.3: Comparison of community- and hospital-acquired pneumonias.

Clinical Findings of Pneumonia

The clinical findings depend on the severity of the infection and underlying cause. Onset can be abrupt or gradual, and is often preceded by upper airway symptoms and associated with malaise, fever, or chills. As the infection progresses cough is established and chest pain and dyspnea can develop.

As the infection progresses expectoration increases and can be purulent or even blood tinged. Mental confusion can arise particularly in elderly or alcoholic patients. If there is multiple lobe involvement then dyspnea can become severe and cyanosis may arise as intrapulmonary shunts become established and more significant. The hypoxemia can be accompanied by hypocapnia as the patient hyperventilates due to the hypoxic drive to breathe.

Chest exams can have variable findings but may include poor respiratory excursion. The consolidated lung fields result in dullness to percussion and a reduction in breath sounds and increase in tactile fremitus. Inspiratory crackles may be heard. With continued progression arterial hypoxia worsens and arterial CO_2 falls due to hyperventilation.

Chest x-ray allows the areas of consolidation to be seen, but typically there is no volume loss, which allows pneumonia to be distinguished from atelectasis (although pneumonia and atelectasis can co-occur). Particularly in the case of a typical pneumonia the complete blood count (CBC) panel will show an elevated white blood cell count. See table 3.4 for summary.

Onset	Progression
Abrupt or gradual	Expectoration—purulent, blood tinged
Upper respiratory symptoms	Mental confusion (elderly or alcoholic patient)
Malaise, chills, fever	Dyspnea and cyanosis with multiple lobe involvement
Cough	Chest exam (variable): - Poor respiratory excursion - Dullness to percussion - Reduced breath sounds - Tactile fremitus (consolidation) - Inspiratory crackles
Chest pain	Opacity on chest x-ray
Dyspnea	No volume loss (distinction from atelectasis)
	Elevated white cell count

Table 3.4: Summary of the clinical findings of pneumonia.

References, Resources, and Further Reading

Text

Farzan, Sattar, with Doris L. Hunsinger and Mary L. Phillips. "Chapter 3." In A *Concise Handbook of Respiratory Diseases*. Reston, VA: Reston Publishing Company, 1978.

Husain, Aliya N. "Chapter 15: The Lung." In *Robbins and Cotran Pathologic Basis of Disease*, 9th ed., edited by Vinay Kumar, Abul K. Abbas, and John C. Aster. Philadelphia: Saunders, an imprint of Elsevier Inc., 2015.

Figures

Figure 3.1: Pathophysiology of acute bronchitis. Grey, Kindred. 2022. CC BY 4.0. https://archive.org/details/3.1_20220203

Figure 3.2: Histological and Radiographic findings for an RSV infection. Grey, Kindred. 2022. CC BY-NC-SA 3.0. Added Giant cells1 by Nephron from WikimediaCommons (CC BY-SA 3.0) and Respiratory syncytial virus by Radswiki, T., et al. from https://doi.org/10.53347/rID-11873 (CC BY-NC-SA 3.0). https://archive.org/details/3.2-new

Figure 3.3: Neutrophils, bacteria, and exudate occupy airspaces in a typical pneumonia. Nephron. 2016. CC BY-SA 3.0. "Acute Pneumonia — Intermed Mag" from WikimediaCommons.

Figure 3.4: General pathophysiology of pneumonia. Grey, Kindred. 2022. CC BY 4.0. https://archive.org/details/3.4_20220203

Table 3.1: Comparison of typical and atypical pneumonia. Includes Case 1 by Bell, D., Hacking, C., et al. from https://doi.org/10.53347/rID-68496 (CC BY-NC-SA 3.0), Acute pneumonia - i — low mag by Nephron from WikimediaCommons (CC BY-SA 3.0), Case 2 by Paks, M., Knipe, H., et al. from https://doi.org/10.53347/rID-27535 (CC BY-NC-SA 3.0), and image 1 by Dr Patsy Lill from University of South Carolina School of Medicine's Microbiologybook.org (Fair use).

Table 3.2: Comparison of bronchopneumonia and lobar pneumonia. Includes Bronchopneumonia by Kindred Grey from Internet archive (CC BY 4.0), Lobar pneumonia by Kindred Grey from Internet archive (CC BY 4.0), X-ray of bronchopneumonia by Franquet T., Chung J.H. from WikimediaCommons (CC BY 4.0), Case 3 by Paks, M., Knipe, H., et al. from https://doi.org/10.53347/rID-26886 (CC BY-NC-SA 3.0).

4. The Restrictive Lung Diseases

Learning objectives

- Relate the signs and symptoms of an interstitial lung disease (ILD) patient to the pathological process of the disease.
- Differentiate between forms of interstitial lung disease via histological appearance and patient history.

Basis of Restrictive Lung Disease

The restrictive lung diseases are characterized by pathophysiological disruption of the lung interstitial tissue that causes problems with lung expansion. As such, these diseases are more specifically referred to as the interstitial lung diseases, or ILDs. There are about 150 conditions that disrupt lung structure and generally produce a restrictive, rather than obstructive, disorder.

This section provides a broad overview and generalized mechanisms of interstitial lung disease. Subclassifications and details of specific conditions are presented in the next section.

Before we start taking about diseases affecting the lung interstitium, let us remind ourselves of what it is.

The interstitial tissue, sometimes referred to as parenchyma, surrounds the alveolar and capillary structures and contributes to the mechanical behavior of the lungs. The interstitium is extremely thin between the alveoli and capillaries, and forms the basement membrane through which gas exchange occurs. On the parenchymal side of the capillaries the interstitium is more substantial and is more involved in fluid exchange. There is also substantial amounts of interstitial tissue in the spaces around major vessels and airways, and it also makes up the interlobular septa.

Mechanisms of ILD

Now we will look at the generalized mechanism of interstitial lung disease (figure 4.1). It is worth noting that the numerous conditions that the term ILD encompasses have subtle differences in mechanism and manifestations, and these differences are what we will deal with elsewhere.

Generally though, ILD starts with an initial insult to the lung (#1, figure 4.1); the type of insult is a major contributor to the different ILD conditions. (It probably will not be what is depicted in figure 4.1, but if it was, it might lead to the inflammatory condition of tiefitis.)

There is then a response by neutrophils and alveolar macrophages (#2, figure 4.1). The macrophage response seems particularly important to the development of ILD. Release of cytokines (#3, figure 4.1) attracts other inflammatory cells, and the arrival of polymorphonuclear leukocytes and lymphocytes play an important role in disease instigation. These cells release cytokines, enzymes, and toxic oxygen radicals that damage and destroy local tissue. Released growth factors, such as TGF-Beta, instigate the transition of mesenchymal cells to fibroblasts.

It is worth noting at this point that some forms of ILD are caused by an exaggerated immune reaction—either through an allergic-like response, or a direct immune disorder.

The destruction of tissue and activity of a growing number of fibroblasts results in the inflamed interstitium becoming fibrosed with excess connective tissue, particularly collagen (#4, figure 4.1).

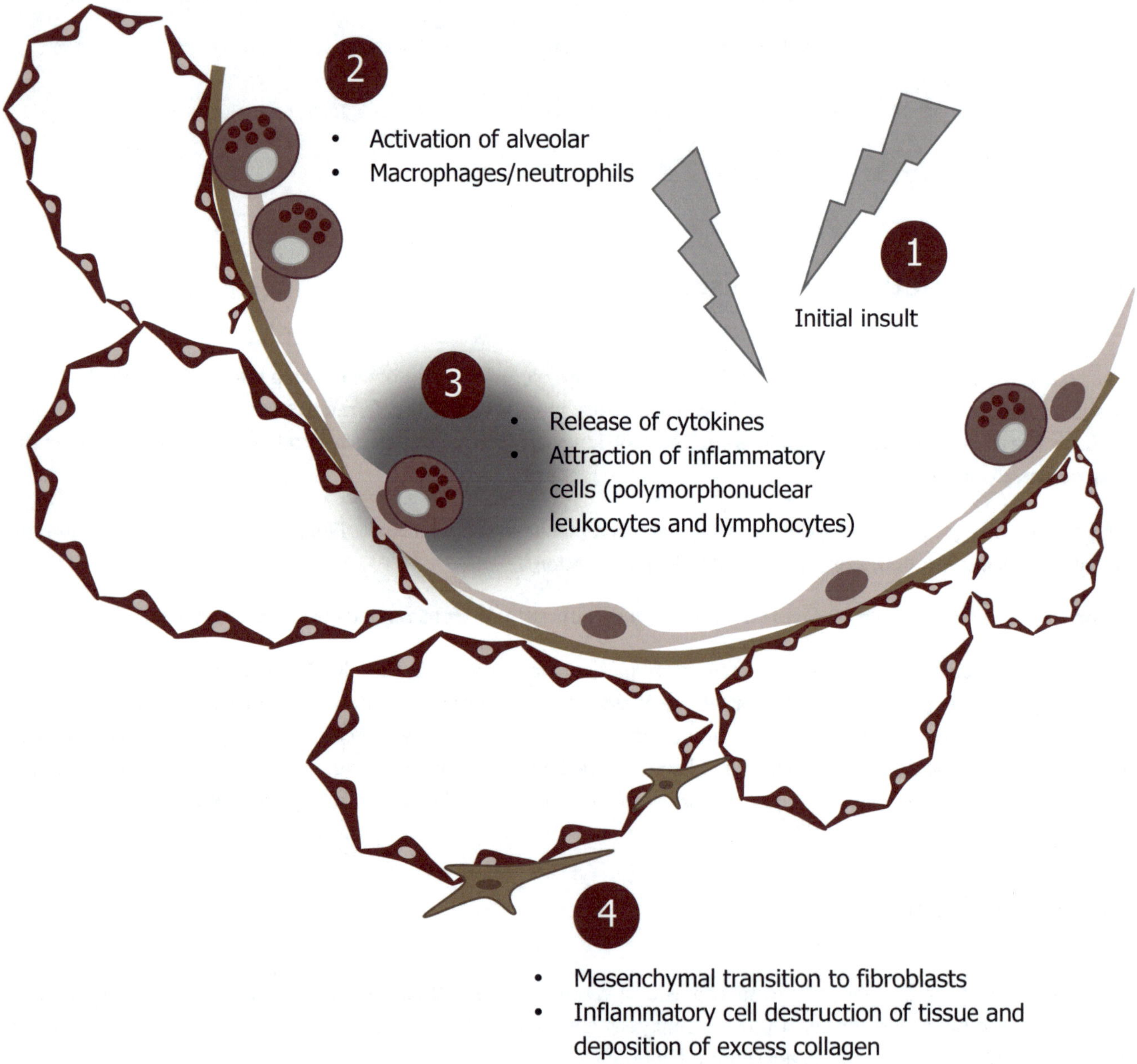

Figure 4.1: Basic mechanism of interstitial lung disease.

Pathology of ILD

These changes in structure dramatically change the functional and mechanical properties of the tissue. The changes also tend to follow a characteristic pattern, although, as you might imagine, different conditions have subtle differences in pattern.

The action of fibroblasts laying down connective tissue, combined with the destruction of alveolar and capillary structures, leads to a widening of airspaces with thick collagenous and infiltrated walls (figure 4.2A and 4.2B), which are a functionally significant departure from the ideal structure for gas exchange.

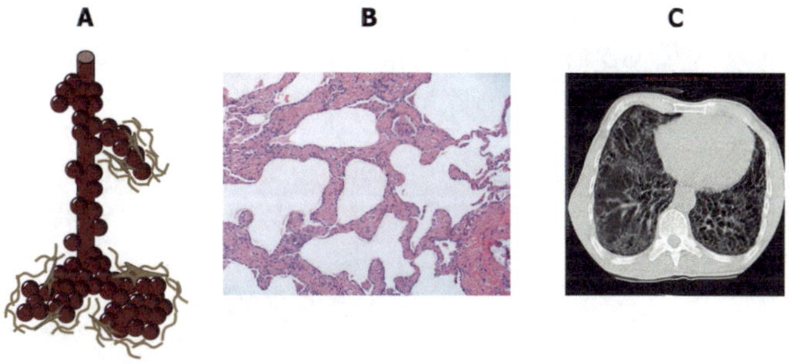

Figure 4.2: Changes in pulmonary histology (A, B) and gross anatomy (C) with interstitial lung disease.

The thickened basement membrane poses a significant obstacle to the transfer of gases, and the dense connective tissue stiffens the lung and thereby reduces its compliance. Combined with loss of capillary beds and airspace surface area, gas exchange is reduced.

At the end of the disease the lung takes on a characteristic honeycomb appearance, and "ground glass opacities" are a hallmark sign on CT images (figure 4.2C). These morphological changes lead to pathophysiological consequences that are shared by most forms of the disease, as all cause varying degrees of interstitial inflammation and connective tissue deposition.

Pathophysiology of ILD

The first major issue is the reduced diffusion capacity of the involved areas, and all ILD patients demonstrate a reduced transfer factor, or DLCO (figure 4.3).

Because of the heterogenous distribution of the disease, and the involvement of the pulmonary circulation, severe V/Q abnormalities arise throughout the lung. This and the reduced diffusion capacity result in hypoxemia. In the chronic disease state this may lead to cor pulmonale (figure 4.3).

The reduction in lung compliance leads to a reduced lung volume. This is easily detected with spirometry as shown by the inner plot of the flow-volume loop in figure 4.3. Because FEV_1 and FVC are both reduced, the ratio frequently remains the same or may even rise; as such FEV_1/FVC is a poor indicator of restrictive disease.

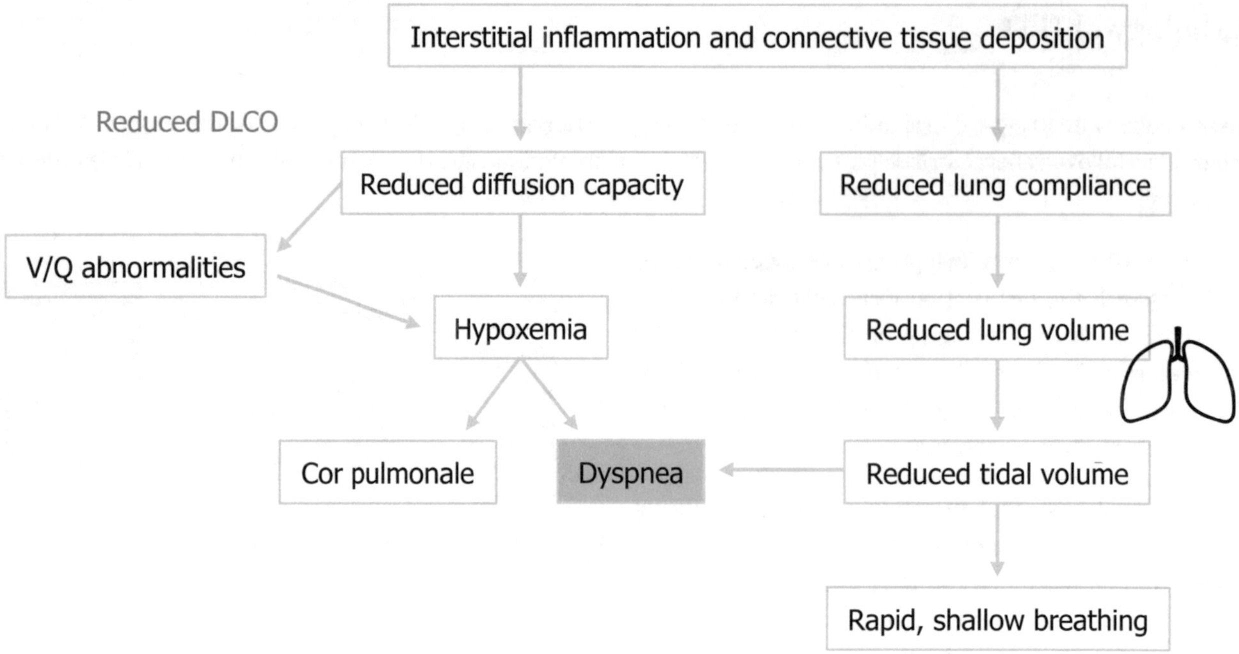

Figure 4.3: Pathophysiological consequences of ILD.

The reduced lung volume and compliance results in a characteristic rapid, shallow breathing pattern as the patient tries to maintain alveolar ventilation (figure 4.3). However, while avoiding unnecessary increases in the work of breathing by not trying to over-expand the noncompliant lung, the rapid shallow breathing proportionally increases dead space ventilation.

The reduction in tidal volume, combined with a raised hypoxic drive to breathe, results in the cardinal symptom of ILD, which is dyspnea (figure 4.3).

Clinical Signs of ILD

The correlation of dyspnea and disease stage is closer in ILD than any other respiratory disease. The onset is insidious, appearing first during exercise, and it likely contributes to the other major complaints of weakness and fatigue. The dyspnea gets progressively worse until it can be debilitating.

Inflammation and excitation of pulmonary receptors leads to a nonproductive and persistent cough, and upon examination patients will have limited chest expansion and demonstrate the characteristic breathing pattern of restrictive lung disease.

Hallmark lung sounds are fine crackles, commonly found at the base of the lung, and may appear louder than expected because of increased transmission through denser than normal tissue.

At later stages of the disease the patient shows signs of the prolonged hypoxemia with digital clubbing and cyanosis.

Forms of Interstitial Lung Disease

The term interstitial lung disease encompasses about 150 different conditions, and the classification of these conditions is amazingly confusing for numerous reasons. Some classifications are developed by "lumpers" who believe the separate conditions are components of the same spectrum of disorders; other classifications are developed by "splitters," who believe the conditions are distinct. This is made more confusing by a lack of consistent nomenclature between disciplines for the same condition—and this spanner in our work starts at the highest classification level, where what pathologists refer to as an interstitial lung disease, radiologists call a diffuse lung disease (figure 4.4). Then of course, we will reduce everything to an acronym just to make it even more fun! Convention will likely become to use the pathologist's nomenclature, but the radiology versions are included here for reference.

Our major subcategory is idiopathic interstitial pneumonia (figure 4.4), or IIP, and this is divided again into six more useful categories that can be distinguished by history, time line, and histological changes. We will deal with these categories in this section, but it might be noted that usual interstitial pneumonia, still frequently called idiopathic pulmonary fibrosis, is the only one that remains untreatable, and early differentiation from the other forms is critical (figure 4.4).

Interstitial lung diseases can also be induced by numerous different environmental causes that produce nuanced conditions that are distinguishable by environmental and social history (figure 4.4) as well as specific histological features.

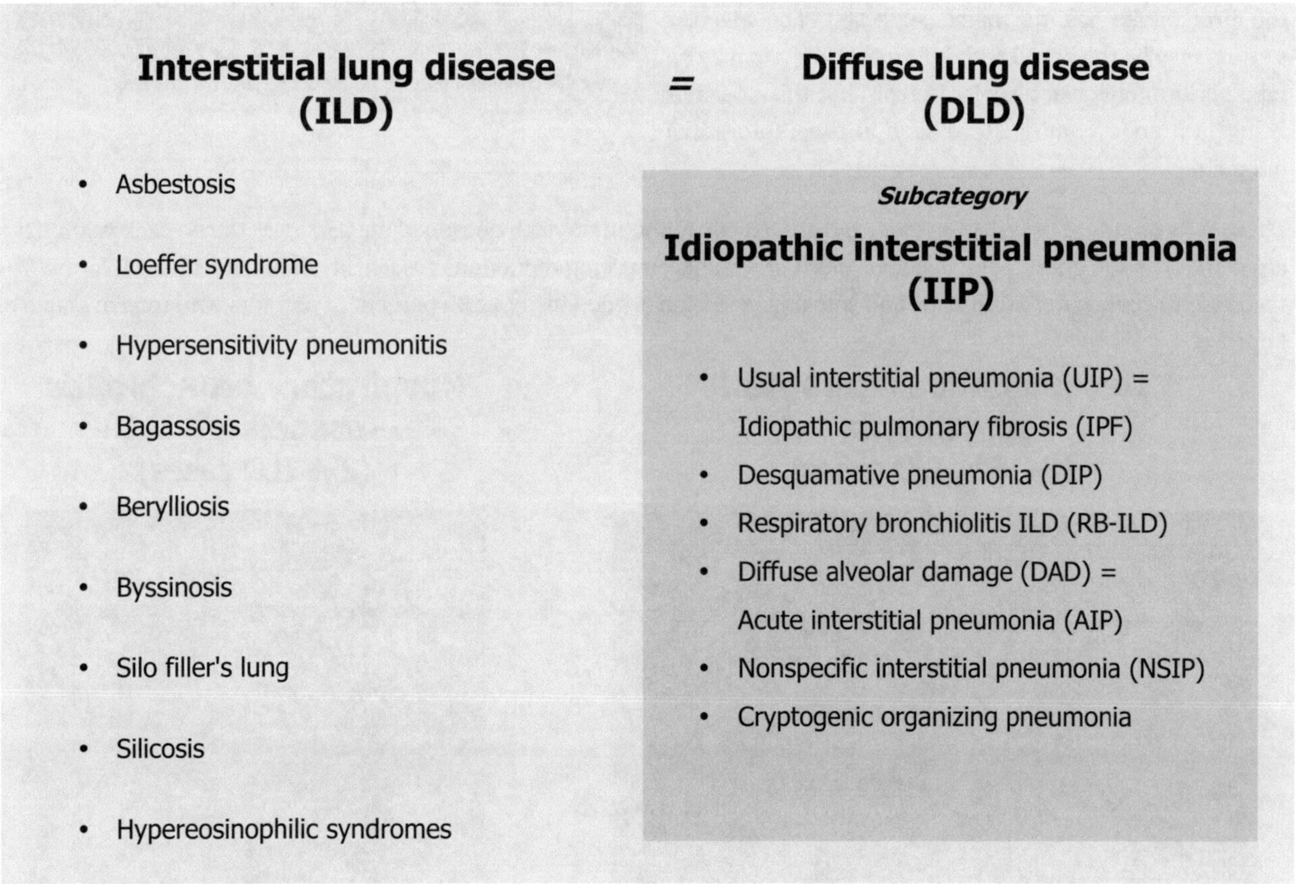

Figure 4.4: Classifications of ILD.

The characteristics of usual interstitial pneumonia have been covered in the "Basis of ILD" section, so let us start looking at the pathophysiological and clinical features of the other broader disease categories.

Desquamative Interstitial Pneumonia and Respiratory Bronchiolitis–Associated ILD

We can deal with the first two together as both share common characteristics and are potentially the same disease occurring in different anatomical locations. Desquamative interstitial pneumonia and respiratory bronchiolitis-associated ILD are both smoking related and are relatively uncommon.

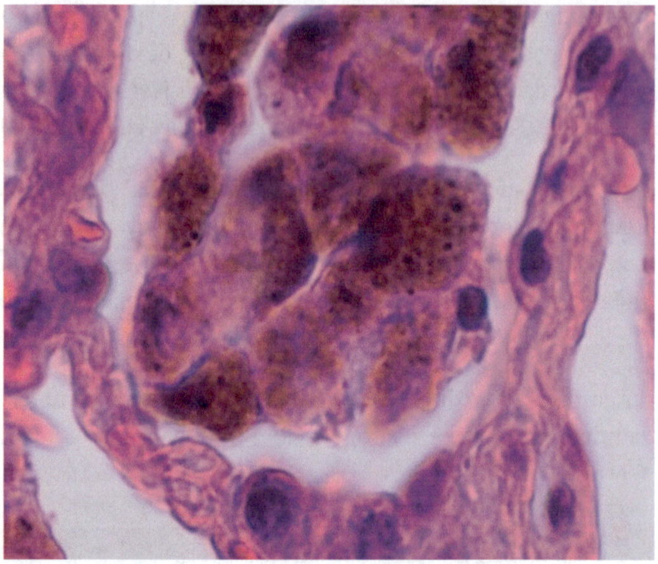

Figure 4.5: Smoker's macrophages occupying an airspace.

The histological hallmark is accumulation of numerous smoker's macrophages in the airspaces (figure 4.5) or the first- and second-order respiratory bronchioles. These macrophages have a characteristic brown pigmentation. In desquamative interstitial pneumonia the airspaces are the primary site of involvement, whereas a respiratory bronchiolitis-associated ILD sees more involvement of the bronchioles (as the name suggests). The alveolar septum may be thickened with infiltrate and there may be mild peribronchilor or alveolar fibrosis, but this does not result in a honeycomb pattern seen in usual interstitial pneumonia.

These ILDs are more prevalent in men, and are usually found in the fifth decade of life and after thirty-pack years. They are marked by the gradual and insidious onset of dyspnea, but lung reductions are usually minimal with both forms. The response to corticosteroid therapy and smoking cessation is good in about 80 percent of patients who remain stable or improve.

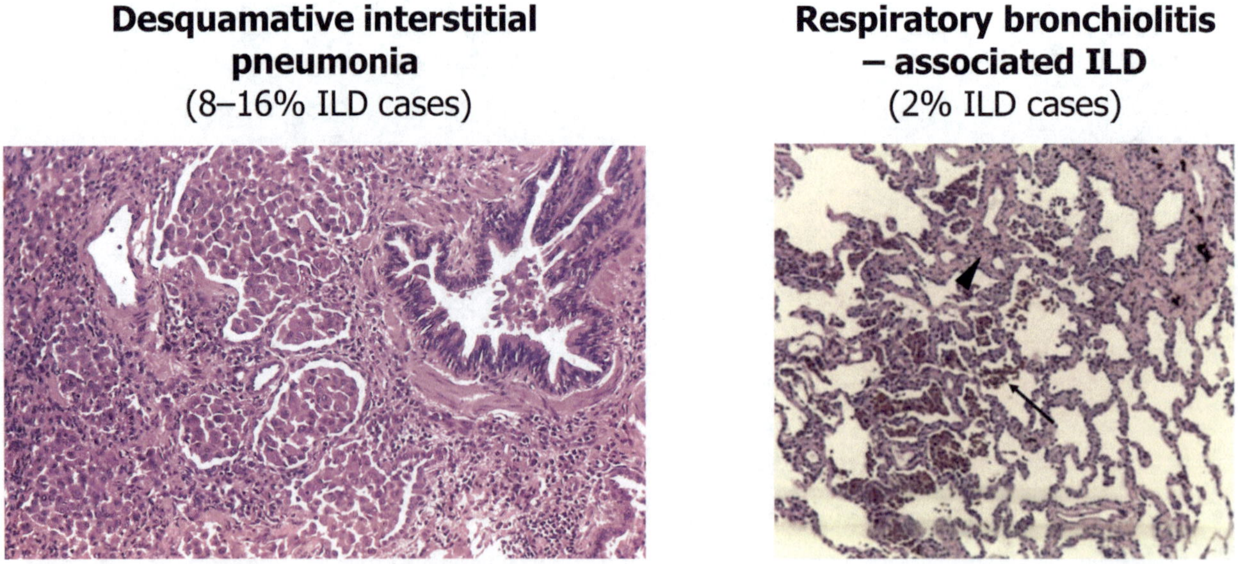

Figure 4.6: Examples of DIP and RB-ILD showing alveolar airspace and bronchiolar involvement in each condition, respectively.

Diffuse Alveolar Damage (DAD)

While the development of most interstitial lung diseases is slow and insidious, the hallmark of diffuse alveolar damage is rapid, occurring in a matter of days and often in previously healthy individuals. The manifestation of the disease is similar to acute respiratory distress syndrome, and in fact it has been suggested that DAD is a form of ARDS.

The start is marked by a brief exudative phase with fluid entering the airspaces, but the following organizing or proliferative phase is what is usually seen by the time a biopsy is taken and where the similarities to ARDS are seen. The alveolar septa are thickened due to the interstitial edema and the septa may collapse or appose each other (figure 4.7). There is marked infiltration of the interstitial and airspaces by inflammatory cells, and type II cells proliferate. The destruction of the alveolar structure leaves a sludgy hyaline membrane of debris. Thrombi in small arteries may also be apparent.

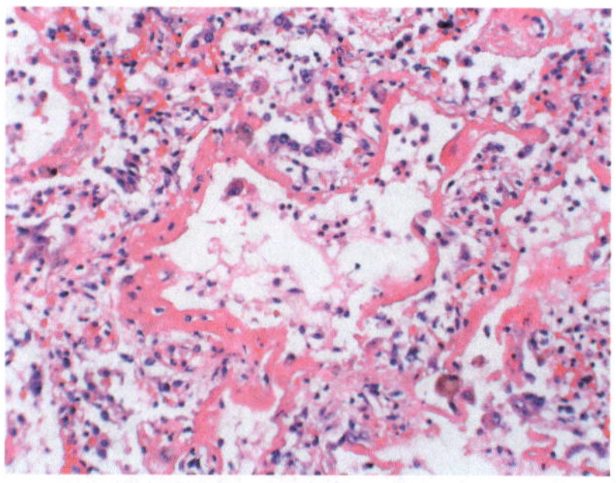

Figure 4.7: Diffuse alveolar damage.

Should the patient survive (about 50 percent do not) the healing phase can show recovery of the alveolar structure with varying degrees of fibrosis. Many patients return to normal lung function, but a few show a progressive fibrotic process that resembles idiopathic pulmonary fibrosis.

Without biopsy, DAD is usually differentiated from other forms of interstitial disease by its rapid onset, but this can be confused with acute exacerbations of other diseases. However, the uniform pattern of damage in real DAD is representative of a single time line.

Nonspecific Interstitial Pneumonia

Our next disease is at least courteous enough to only have one name, nonspecific interstitial pneumonia (NSIP), but irritatingly, it has three groups that are determined by the degree of either interstitial inflammation or fibrosis. Group 1 is primarily inflammation, group 2 involves inflammation and fibrosis, and group 3 is primarily fibrosis. The differences in groups are most clearly seen looking at the extremes—group 1 shows the puffy alveolar septa infiltrated with lymphocytes (left panel, figure 4.8), whereas group 3 shows a matrix of fibrosis that can be distinguished from usual interstitial pneumonia by the absence of fibroblastic foci and a homogenous onset and distribution (right panel, figure 4.8). As its name suggests, the distinguishing feature of nonspecific interstitial pneumonia is the lack of features that determine it to be something else. If that sounds a bit wishy-washy, take solace in the fact that even experts argue over its classification.

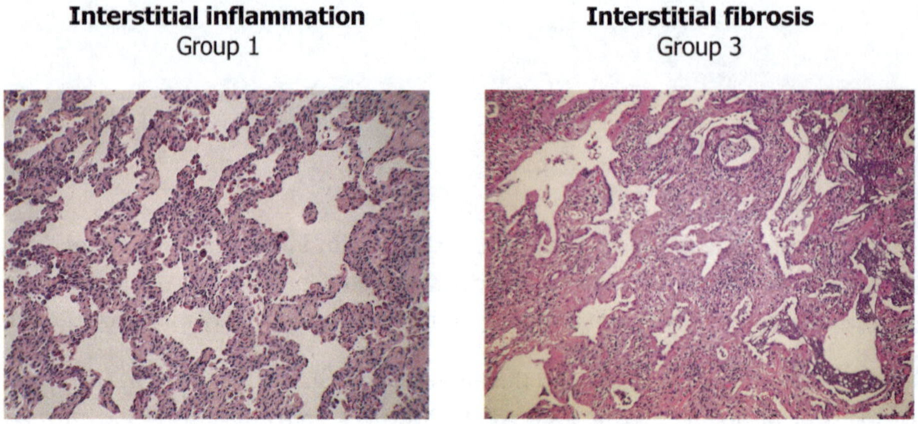

Figure 4.8: Extremes of nonspecific interstitial pneumonia.

The presence of lymphocytes in biopsy and bronchoalveolar lavage fluid suggests the involvement of the immune system in the pathogenesis of nonspecific interstitial pneumonia. This is supported by the occurrence of NSIP in immune diseases such as HIV infection and several connective tissue disorders including polymyositis, rheumatoid arthritis, and systemic sclerosis. Our understanding of the pathological mechanisms is still evolving.

Cryptogenic Organizing Pneumonia

Our final major classification is cryptogenic organizing pneumonia (COP). This form of interstitial disease affects the distal bronchioles, respiratory bronchioles, and alveoli, but the primary site of injury is usually the alveolar walls.

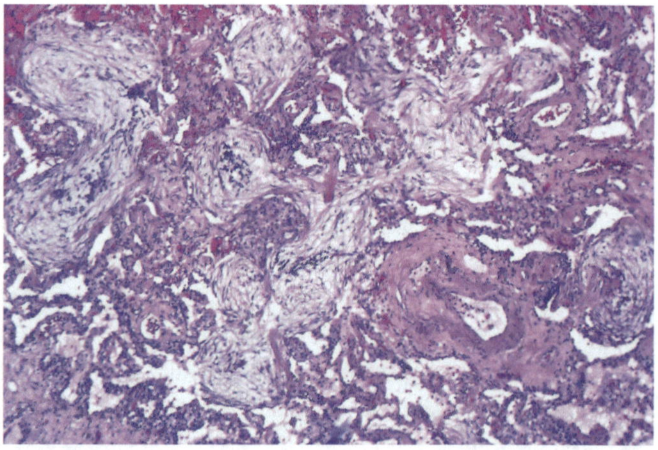

Figure 4.9: Distal airways affected by COP showing butterfly-shaped fibrotic lesions.

The hallmark of COP is an excessive proliferation of granulation tissue made of collagen-embedded fibroblasts and myofibroblasts that starts in the alveolar space. These plugs of fibrotic tissue may extend from one alveolus to another via the pores of Kohn and give rise to a characteristic butterfly pattern. The pathogenesis is an initial alveolar injury, with plasma proteins leaking into the alveolar lumen that is followed by recruited fibroblasts depositing connective tissue with the lumen itself. These fibrotic lesions show a homogenous time line and movement to the distal airways, but are actually reversible, which is in contrast of the lesions seen in usual interstitial pneumonia. In COP the lung architecture is maintained, probably through more thorough regulation of angiogenesis and apoptosis than that seen in usual interstitial pneumonia (UIP).

The onset of COP is marked with dyspnea and dry cough (as with most ILDs), and it has a moderate time line of a couple of months, after which symptoms subside. History is again important to determine the initial insult, and potential culprits include connective tissue disease, new medications, or exposure to therapeutic radiation, fumes, or dusts.

Environment-Induced ILDs

Now we will look at several specific forms of interstitial disease that are related to occupational exposure. While these forms of ILD have some distinguishing factors, the importance of taking a good history cannot be understated.

Silicosis

Silicosis is related to exposure to silica that occurs frequently in occupations such as stone cutting, foundry work, and mining. Cutting or breaking stone can produce crystalline silica, and when less than 5 microns in diameter, it becomes respirable. When particle size is between 1 and 3 microns, it can reach the alveoli.

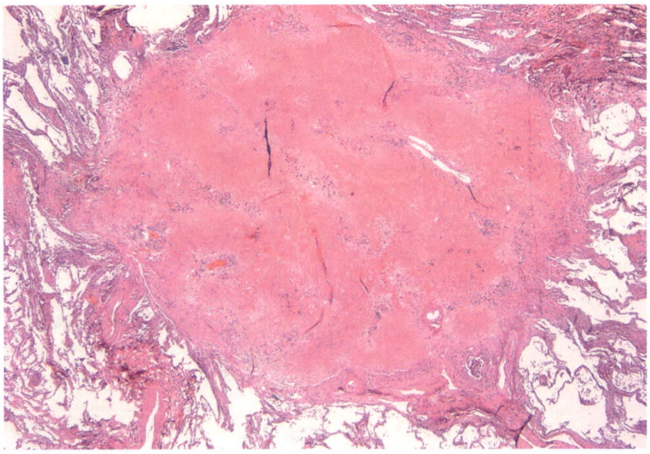

Figure 4.10: Silicotic nodule in the parenchyma of the lung.

The formation of silicosis can be acute with heavy brief exposure (often seen in sandblasters), or chronic and insidious with more prolonged lighter exposures. The process is initiated with alveolar macrophages engulfing the crystals. In response they release cytokines to attract lymphocytes, neutrophils, and fibroblasts—and a familiar story of tissue destruction and laying down of collagen begins. (You might note at this point that engulfing silica in vitro has been shown to damage macrophages, causing them to release their intracellular enzymes, which may contribute to the destructive mechanism in vivo.)

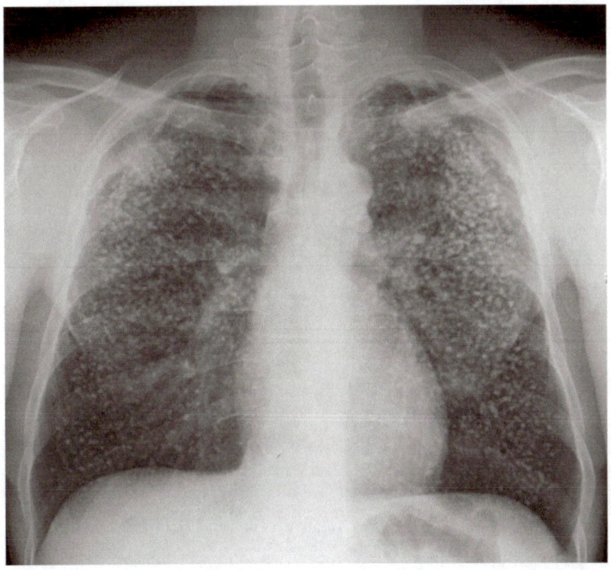

Figure 4.11: Silicotic nodules distributed throughout the lungs.

The pattern of collagen deposition is distinct, with silicotic nodules forming with concentric fibers producing a whirled pattern (figure 4.10). These nodules are distributed throughout the lung but are more common in the upper lobes and perihilar area (figure 4.11). They tend to be surrounded by distorted lung tissue that may show emphysematous changes. Ongoing disease coalescence of the nodules produces irregular masses of noncaseating granulomas. This progressive massive fibrosis can be helped with concurrent TB or atypical mycobacterial disease where caseating granulomas may also be present. Likewise silicosis may impair the macrophage response to TB. It causes contraction of the upper lobes and may lead to emphysema in the lower lobes, sometimes with large bullous changes. The pathophysiology of silicosis is summarized in figure 4.12.

After an insidious, asymptomatic beginning, the main symptom of silicosis is dyspnea, with or without cough (cough is likely generated by concurrent smoking). The dyspnea is progressive but other symptoms that occur are often due to secondary, superimposed infection making repeated bacteriological studies important.

The pathophysiology of silicosis is summarized in figure 4.12.

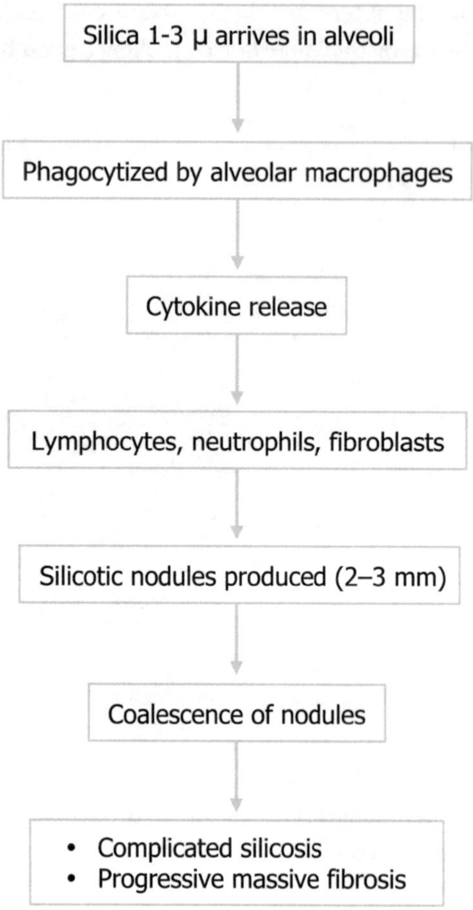

Figure 4.12: The pathophysiology of silicosis.

Asbestosis

There are a number of pulmonary manifestations arising from exposure to asbestos. Previously used in the construction and manufacturing industries, the occurrence of related illness led to legislation to restrict its use. However, demolition or renovation of asbestos-containing buildings can still lead to air-born asbestos exposure. The pulmonary manifestations include pulmonary fibrosis, bronchogenic carcinoma, pleural effusion, pleural fibrosis, and mesothelioma. We will deal with the pulmonary fibrosis here and what is known as asbestosis.

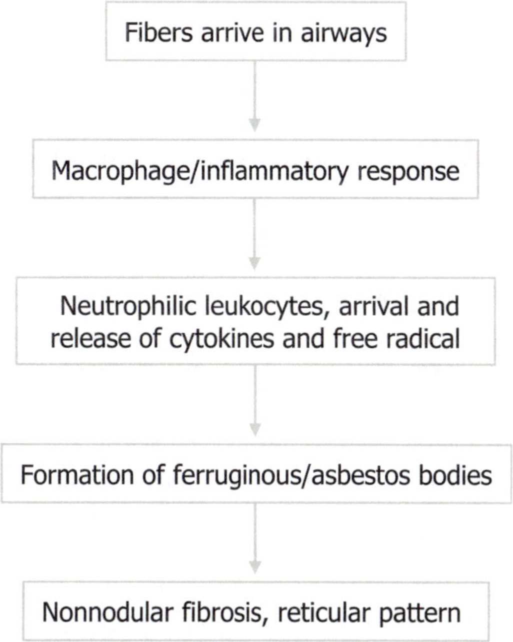

Figure 4.13: Pathophysiology of asbestosis.

The disease course (summarized in figure 4.13) is similar to that described for silicosis. Asbestos fibers arrive in the alveoli and macrophages initiate an inflammatory response. Note that the arrival of neutrophilic leukocytes and their release of cytokines and oxygen radicals seem to play a significant role. Short fibers can be phagocytized and removed, but larger fibers persist in the airway and perpetuate the inflammatory reaction, promoting fibrosis.

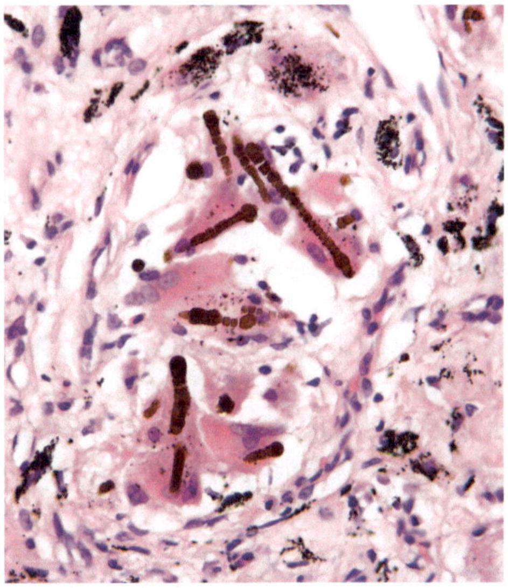

Figure 4.14: Ferruginous bodies associated with asbestosis.

Histologically, these fibers can been seen as asbestos bodies, or ferruginous bodies, as they are coated with iron-containing protein (figure 4.14).

Fibrosis ensues, but in contrast to silicosis, asbestos-related fibrosis is nonnodular and mostly involves the lower lung fields and frequently includes pleural thickening.

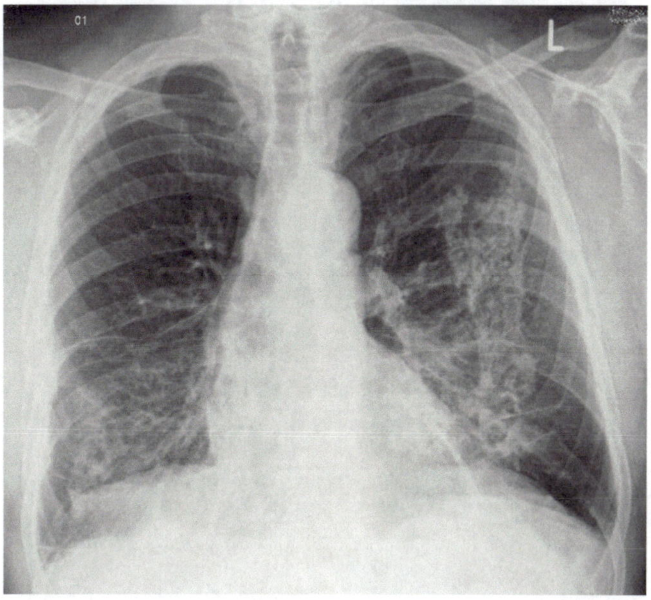

Figure 4.15: Radiographic findings in asbestosis.

The extent of fibrosis is highly variable, from thickened alveolar septum to complete destruction of the alveolar spaces. In the advanced disease honeycomb lung can be observed with CT. Radiography of later-stage disease shows reticular interstitial markings in the lower lung fields (left panel, figure 4.15). Pleural changes are also more common. Rounded atelectasis may occur after a pleural effusion has been reabsorbed and caused a section of the airway to become trapped. A rounded atelectasis is indicated by the arrow in figure 4.15, and care should be taken not to mistake this for a neoplasm. Abestosis is a risk factor for the development of mesothelioma and should be considered for patients working in "at-risk" environments or occupations.

Coal worker's pneumoconiosis (CWP)

CWP arises after prolonged exposure to coal dust. While drilling through rock the miner may be susceptible to silicosis, but prolonged and heavy exposure to aerosolized carbon (that is not usually fibrogenic in lesser exposures) can result in its own distinct condition. Even then it can take ten to twelve years of underground exposure to develop.

Again we see the process start with phagocytosis of the coal dust by macrophages after the mucocillary escalator is overwhelmed. The macrophages launch their inflammatory process, and tissue damage is caused by the resultant cytokine bloom and oxygen radical and enzyme release. Fibroblasts form reticulin networks, but there is no significant collagen deposition. Aggregates of reticulin fibers, macrophages, and dust form coal macules (figure 4.16). The coal macules appear as black spots in lung sections and give rise to the condition's nickname of "black lung."

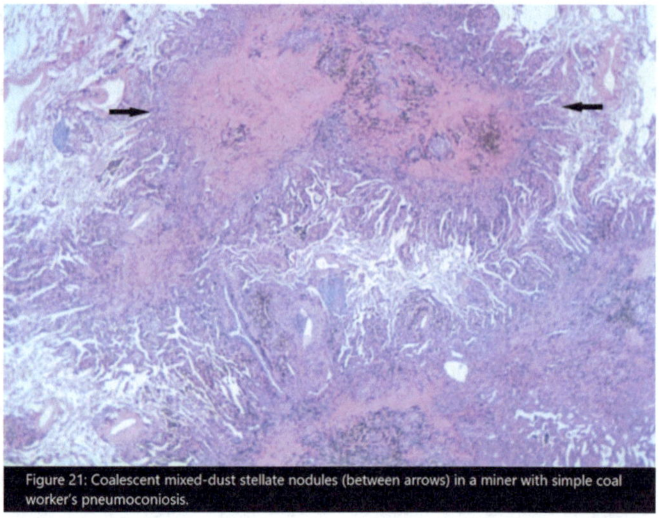

Figure 4.16: Example of coal macules in simple CWP showing fibrosis and coal macules.

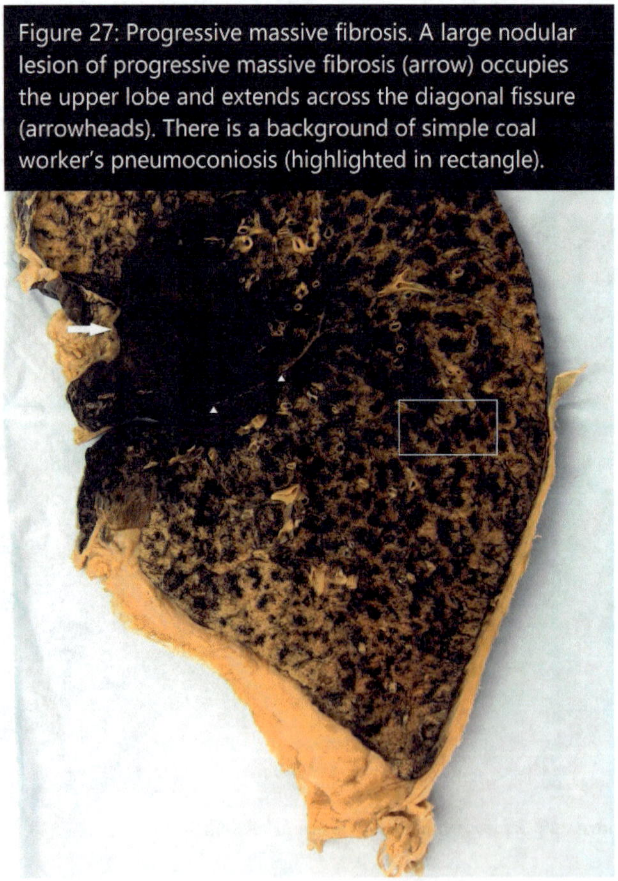

Figure 4.17: Large perihilar lesion in complicated CWP.

The coal macules are associated with dilation of the respiratory bronchioles that can manifest as focal centrilobar emphysema (figure 4.16). This is referred to as simple CWP, whereas the less common, complicated form involves progressive massive fibrosis, usually in the upper lobes, as in silicosis. However, in CWP these lesions are black and relatively homogenous, where as in silicosis they are a conglomeration of intersecting nodules. Figure 4.17 shows a large black fibrotic lesion destroying the perihilar lung parenchyma.

Clinical manifestations are often complicated by concurrent cigarette smoking that may alone explain the frequency of chronic bronchitis in CWP patients. The simple form can be asymptomatic, but the complicated form produces dyspnea and signs of respiratory failures, pulmonary hypertension, and cor pulmonale.

Berylliosis

The last occupational disorder we will look at is berylliosis, or chronic beryllium disease (CBD), that occurs after exposure to beryllium, a metal used in manufacturing. Here the start to our story is a little different. Beryllium arrives in the airway and there is a hypersensitization of T cells. On subsequent exposures the T cells proliferate—the bronchoalveolar lavage (BAL) fluid of berylliosis patients is rich in sensitized CD4+ cells.

Now we return to our pattern: the abundant CD4+ cells release proinflammatory cytokines and granulomatous fibrosis occurs (figure 4.18). The granulomas (figure 4.19) are indistinguishable from those caused by sarcoidosis (which are also caused by CD4+ cells), and many CBD patients may be misdiagnosed as sarcoidosis cases, so appropriate history taking is paramount. Usually CBD involves greater interstitial inflammation, but the most definitive diagnosis comes from the beryllium lymphocyte proliferation test. The test involves exposing lymphocytes from the patient's blood or BAL fluid to different concentrations of beryllium and assaying their proliferation.

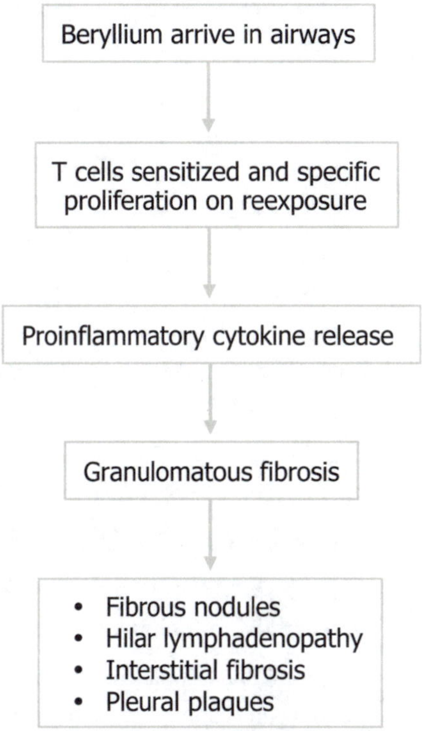

Figure 4.18: Pathophysiology of berylliosis.

Susceptibility to becoming hypersensitized appears to have a significant genetic component. Why the process continues after exposure has stopped is unclear, but possibilities include a fundamental T cell disorder, or the fact that the insoluble beryllium causes apoptosis of macrophages, leading them to release a previously phagocytized beryllium load.

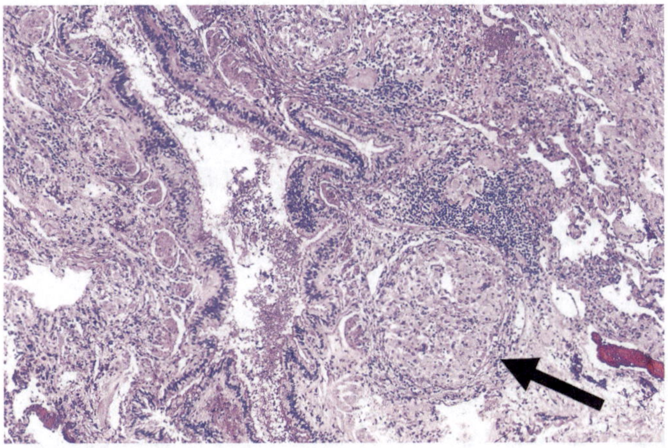
Figure 4.19: Granulomas of berylliosis.

As the disease progresses, radiographic findings show that the granuoles can become more organized to produce fibrous nodules that may begin to impact lung function. The immune system involvement can produce hilar lymphadenopathy, and common later signs include interstital fibrosis and pleural thickening.

Summary

So there is a selection of interstitial lung diseases that, while sharing the pathophysiological manifestations of restrictive lung disease, can be distinguished through good history taking or identifying distinct histological features.

References, Resources, and Further Reading

Text

Farzan, Sattar, with Doris L. Hunsinger and Mary L. Phillips. "Chapters 12–15." In A *Concise Handbook of Respiratory Diseases*. Reston, VA: Reston Publishing Company, 1978.

Husain, Aliya N. "Chapter 15: The Lung." In *Robbins and Cotran Pathologic Basis of Disease*, 9th ed., edited by Vinay Kumar, Abul K. Abbas, and John C. Aster. Philadelphia: Saunders, an imprint of Elsevier Inc., 2015.

Figures

Figure 4.1: Basic mechanism of interstitial lung disease. Grey, Kindred. 2022. CC BY 4.0. https://archive.org/details/4.1_20220203

Figure 4.2: Changes in Pulmonary histology (A, B) and gross anatomy (C) with interstitial lung disease. Grey, Kindred. 2022. CC BY-NC-SA 3.0. Added Sphere by Ates Evren Aydinel from Noun Project (CC BY 3.0), Smoking-related interstitial fibrosis – Case 268 by Yale Rosen from Flickr (CC BY-SA 2.0), and Case 1 by Jones, J., Weerakkody, Y., et al. from https://doi.org/10.53347/rID-14479 (CC BY-NC-SA 3.0). https://archive.org/details/4.2_20220203

Figure 4.3: Pathophysiological consequences of ILD. Grey, Kindred. 2022. CC BY 4.0. Added Lungs by regara from Noun Project (CC BY 3.0). https://archive.org/details/4.3_20220203

Figure 4.4: Classifications of ILD. Grey, Kindred. 2022. CC BY 4.0. https://archive.org/details/4.4_20220203

Figure 4.5: 'Smoker's macrophages occupying an airspace. Häggström, Mikael. 2021. Public domain. From WikimediaCommons.

Figure 4.6: Examples of DIP and RB-ILD showing alveolar airspace and bronchiolar involvement in each condition respectively. Grey, Kindred. 2022. CC BY-SA 2.0. Added Desquamative interstitial pneumonia by Yale Rosen from Flickr (CC BY-SA 2.0) and Histopathology of respiratory bronchiolitis by Sousa, C., Rodrigues, M., Carvalho, A. et al. from WikimediaCommons (CC BY 4.0). https://archive.org/details/4.6_20220203

Figure 4.7: Diffuse alveolar damage. Rosen, Yale. 2009. CC BY-SA 2.0. From WikimediaCommons.

Figure 4.8: Extremes of non-specific interstitial pneumonia. Grey, Kindred. 2022. Added Non-specfic interstitial pneumonia (NSIP), cellular variant Case 137 by Yale Rosen from Flickr (CC BY-SA 2.0) and Non-specfic interstitial pneumonia (NSIP), fibrosing variant Case 138 by Yale Rosen from Flickr (CC BY-SA 2.0). https://archive.org/details/4.8_20220203

Figure 4.9: Distal airways effected by COP showing butterfly-shaped fibrotic lesions. Rosen, Yale. 2010. CC BY-SA 2.0. From Flickr.

Figure 4.10: Silicotic nodule in parenchyma of lung. Rosen, Yale. 2012. CC BY-SA 2.0. From WikimediaCommons.

Figure 4.11: Silicotic nodules in right upper lobe indicated by arrows. Radswiki, T., Weerakkody, Y., et al. 2020. CC BY-NC-SA 3.0. Case 12 from https://doi.org/10.53347/rID-12513.

Figure 4.12: The pathophysiology of silicosis. Grey, Kindred. 2022. CC BY 4.0. https://archive.org/details/4.12_20220203

Figure 4.13: Pathophysiology of asbestosis. Grey, Kindred. 2022. CC BY 4.0. https://archive.org/details/4.13_20220203

Figure 4.14: Ferrugenous bodies associated with asbestosis. Nephron. 2009. CC BY-SA 3.0. From WikimediaCommons.

Figure 4.15: Radiographic finding in asbestosis. Weerakkody, Y., et al. 2021. CC BY-NC-SA 3.0. "Case 4" from https://doi.org/10.53347/rID-7465.

Figure 4.16: Example of Coal Macules in simple CWP. CDC. 2020. Public domain. Figure 21 from CDC.

Figure 4.17: Large peri-hilar lesion in complicated CWP. CDC. 2020. Public domain. Figure 27 from CDC.

Figure 4.18: Pathophysiology of berylliosis. Grey, Kindred. 2022. CC BY 4.0. https://archive.org/details/4.19_20220203

Figure 4.19: Granulomas of berylliosis. Rosen, Yale. 2012. CC BY-SA 2.0. From WikimediaCommons.

5. Acute Respiratory Distress Syndrome

Learning objectives

- Describe the pathogenesis and pathophysiology of acute respiratory distress syndrome (ARDS).

Before consensus on its name was reached in 1992, acute respiratory distress syndrome, or ARDS, was known by numerous names, such as "shock lung," "wet lung syndrome," "white lung syndrome," and "congestive atelectasis." These examples of previous names tell you something about ARDS:

1. that it has multiple causes, and
2. when we see the words "shock," "wet," "congestive," and "white" (in reference to its radiological appearance, figure 5.8), there are likely inflammatory and edema components.

So let us look at the pathophysiological processes underlying what is now universally known as ARDS.

Pathology of ARDS

There are about two hundred thousand cases of ARDS in the United States each year. Each case starts with an initial insult to the lung parenchyma and there are numerous examples of this instigating event, but the most common of these (and therefore worth remembering) are **sepsis**, **pulmonary aspiration**, and **thoracic trauma**. The insult can arrive from the airway, such as in pulmonary aspiration or smoke inhalation, or can arrive from the bloodstream, as in a fat embolism or blood-born pathogen.

Regardless of the insult's route or indeed form, the ensuing pathological events are similar and lead to the same alteration of the lungs. What is initiated is a defensive inflammatory response, and what results is vascular endothelial and alveolar epithelial damage and a leaky alveolar capillary membrane.

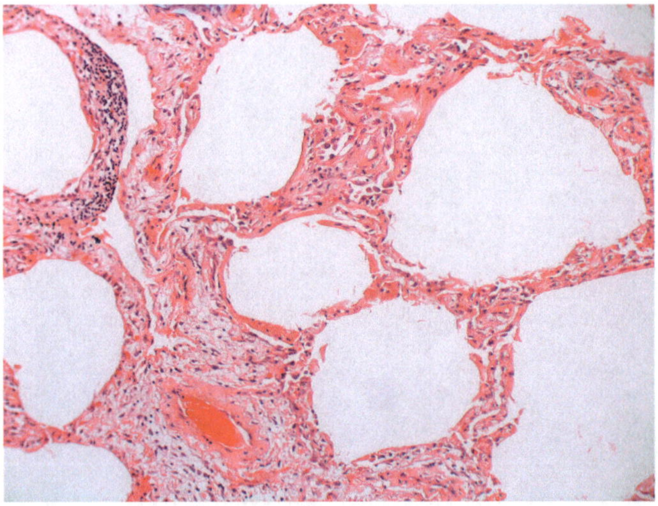

Figure 5.1: The inflammatory response of ARDS causes a blockade of pulmonary vasculature (see in the clot formed in the vessel, bottom left).

Let us look at the process step-by-step.

1. The insult (whatever the form) causes diffuse alveolar damage that includes some alveolar septal thickening, hyperplasia of pneumocytes, and formation of eosinophilic hyaline membranes. Despite its name, this "membrane" is not an organized s, purposeful structure, but should be thought of as accumulating debris that is going to block gas exchange.
2. The injury causes release of inflammatory cytokines, and tumor necrosis factor, interleukin (IL)-1, IL-6, and IL-8 have been shown to be particularly involved in ARDS.
3. The cytokines attract neutrophils to the area, and polymorphonuclear neutrophils play a central role in the inflammatory process. Other cell types can also arrive, such as macrophages, lymphocytes, and fibroblasts, and there is also activation of coagulation and the complement system. Some of the small vessels can be completely obliterated by fibrin-platelet aggregation (figure 5.1), and early proliferation of fibroblasts starts the process of fibrous tissue formation.
4. The neutrophils, however, begin to release toxic mediators, but rather than resolve the underlying, initial problem, the released reactive oxygen species and proteases disrupt the capillary endothelium and the alveolar epithelium.
5. With these barriers compromised, protein escapes into the interstitial tissue and water follows, and then the compromised alveolar wall can be breached and water enters the airspace.
6. Along with water cellular debris and proteins that accumulate in the airspace, providing an oncotic force to draw more water into the airspace, this cellular junk can settles and adds to the hyaline membrane to coat the inner surface of the alveolus, forming a barrier to gas exchange that will persist even after the edema has been resolved.

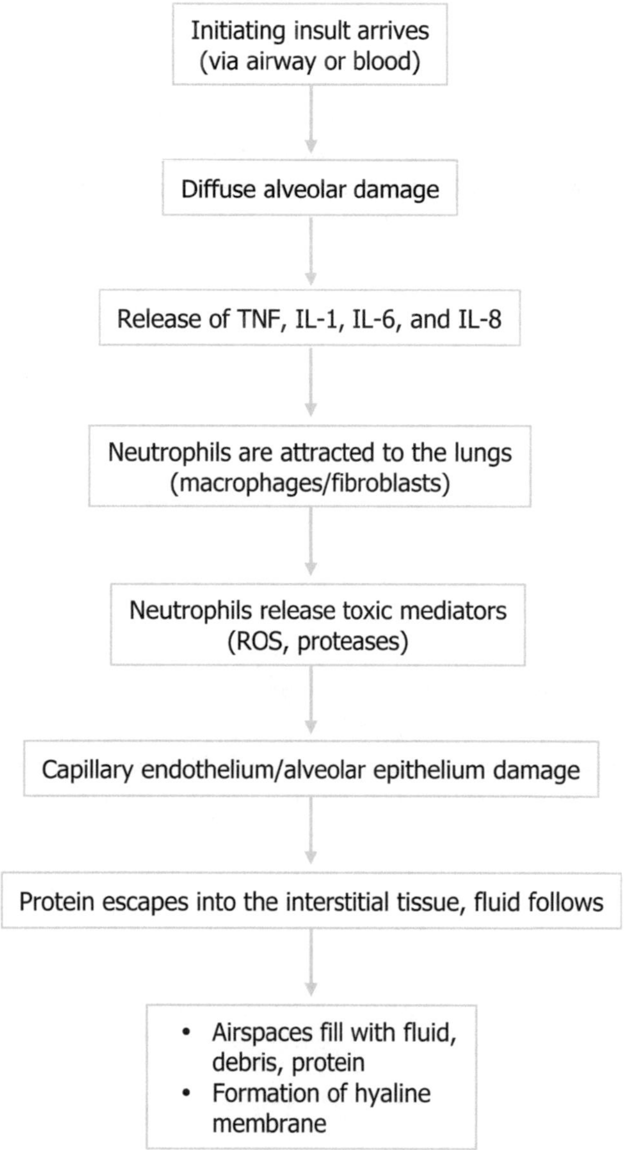

Figure 5.2: Pathophysiological events of ARDS. ROS = reactive oxygen species.

The process is summarized in figure 5.2.

Stages of ARDS

There are three defined stages for the progression of ARDS.

1. **Exudative:** The first six to seven days comprise the exudative phase that begins with edema appearing in the interstitial walls seen here by the widened alveolar septum. Cellular debris can also be seen in the airspaces, and this can continue with the formation of the hyaline membranes that coat the alveolar surface (figure 5.3).

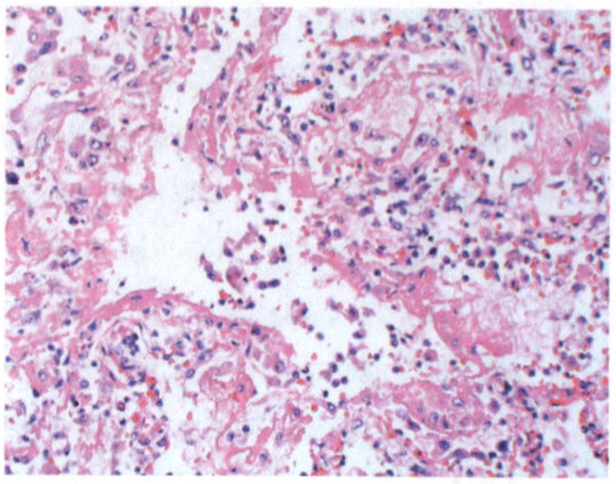

Figure 5.3: Alveolar wall edema and onset of hyaline membrane formation during the exudative phase of ARDS. The debris inside the airspace is the result of the inflammatory response and the beginning of a hyaline membrane made of "cellular debris."

2. **Proliferative:** In the early proliferative stage, there is increased cell infiltration and squamous metaplasia with proliferation of type II cells (figure 5.4), and these mitotic type II cells have a "hob-nail" like appearance over a time line of weeks. The infiltrating cells include fibroblasts that begin laying down collagen.

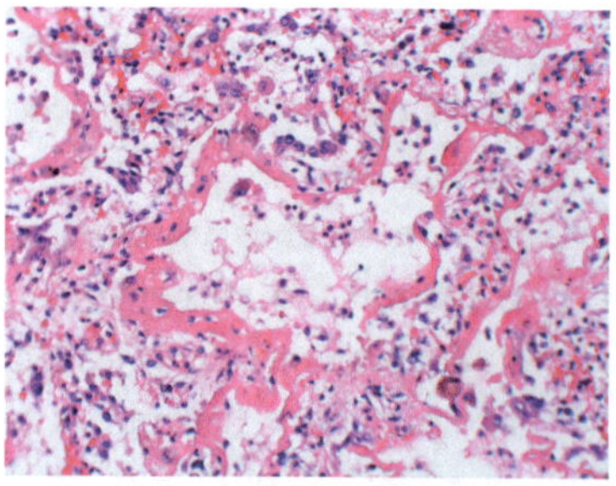

Figure 5.4: Proliferation of type II cells and infiltration of fibroblasts in the proliferative phase of ARDS. A clear amount of debris in the airspace can be seen and forms a hyaline membrane that will impede gas exchange.

3. **Fibrotic:** Without resolution the patient may enter the third stage, fibrotic stage, that occurs over months (figure 5.5). This stage occurs much later and is a consequence of unresolved chronic inflammation. Diffuse fibrosis permanently obliterates normal lung architecture and may form cysts.

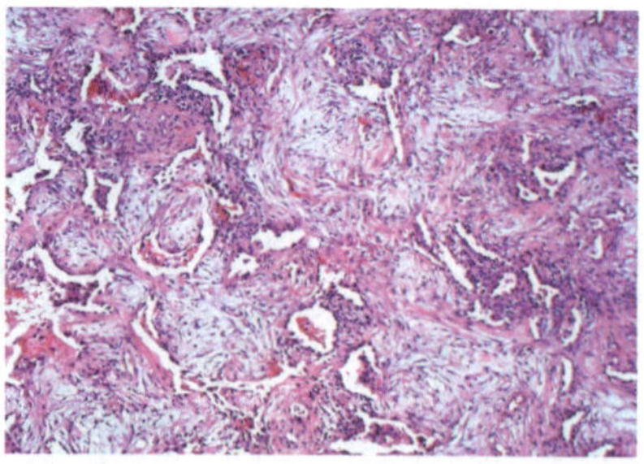

Figure 5.5: Fibrotic stage of ARDS.

Systemic pathophysiology of ARDS

We start with initial lung injury leading to alveolarcapillary leaking. As we have seen, this leads to the airspace edema and hyaline membrane formation.

The lack of gas exchange from affected areas produces a right-left shunt and hypoxemia will result. This produces dyspnea, the major symptom of ARDS.

But the disruption caused by the inflammatory process also leads to other pathophysiological issues. The loss of type II cells causes surfactant production to decline. This of course reduces lung compliance, and the resultant increase in the work of breathing contributes to the patient's dyspnea.

But we are still not done. The fibrin clots forming obstructions in the lung microvasculature lead to V/Q mismatches, and these contribute to the hypoxemia. The obstructed vasculature also produces pulmonary hypertension, which is exacerbated by the vasculature's response to the hypoxia.

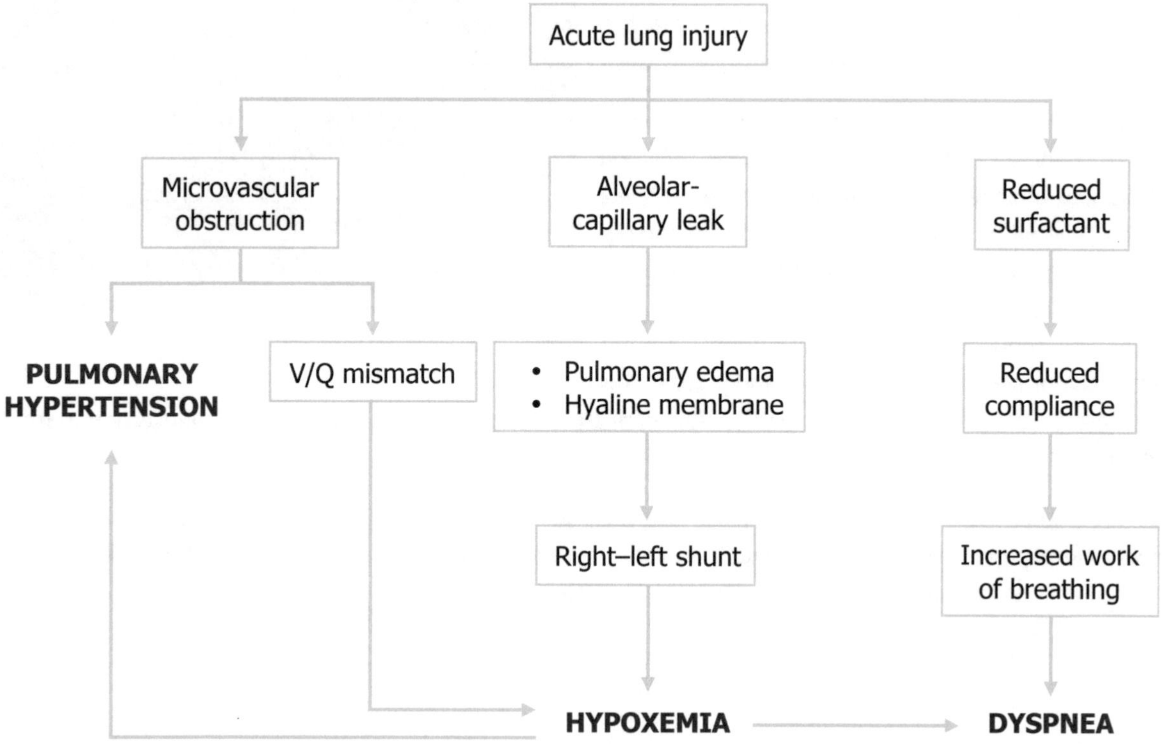

Figure 5.6: Pathophysiology of ARDS.

These mechanisms are reflected in the clinical manifestations of ARDS.

Clinical signs of ARDS

The onset of dyspnea usually occurs within one to two days after the initial injury, and as tachypnea arises, this symptom progressively worsens. Cough is common and may produce blood-tinged sputum. Findings on chest exam may be surprisingly scant, but some bronchial breath sounds and crackles may be heard.

As cyanosis becomes apparent, minute ventilation and dyspnea continue to increase and the patient will likely become distressed.

A high ventilatory rate driven by the hypoxemia can produce hypocapnia and a respiratory alkalosis. The arterial pH can be complicated by the underlying disorder, and it is not uncommon for a mixed acid–base disorder to occur with concurrent respiratory alkalosis and metabolic acidosis. At the onset of respiratory failure arterial CO_2 will rise and produce a respiratory acidosis.

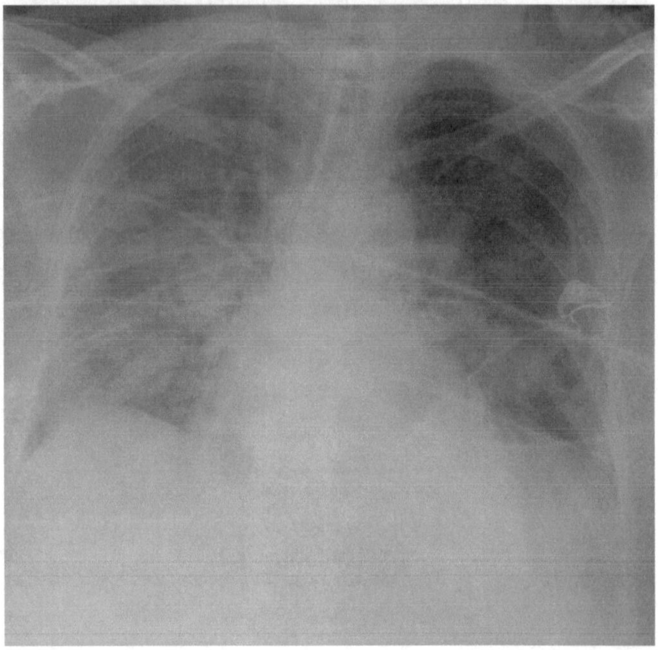

Figure 5.7: Diffuse bilateral densities associated with ARDS.

Radiographic findings are an essential part of diagnosing the ARDS patient and will show diffuse bilateral interstitial and airspace densities caused by the edema (figure 5.7). Normal heart and vessel size and absence of pleural effusion distinguish ARDS from cardiogenic pulmonary edema. Although the x-ray gives the appearance of diffuse edema, high-resolution CT often shows that the process is heterogeneous and patchy. This heterogeneity is reflected by remnant patchy fibrosis if the patient recovers; however, the mortality rate for ARDS is around 50 percent.

So now you should have a clear understanding that after an initial insult to the lung an exaggerated and perpetual inflammatory response leads to the destruction of the alveolar–capillary interface. The resulting edema and hyaline membrane formation produces severe hypoxemia and a critically ill patient.

References, Resources, and Further Reading

Text

Farzan, Sattar, with Doris L. Hunsinger and Mary L. Phillips. "Chapter 27." In A *Concise Handbook of Respiratory Diseases*. Reston, VA: Reston Publishing Company, 1978.

Husain, Aliya N. "Chapter 15: The Lung." In *Robbins and Cotran Pathologic Basis of Disease*, 9th ed., edited by Vinay Kumar, Abul K. Abbas, and John C. Aster. Philadelphia: Saunders, an imprint of Elsevier Inc., 2015.

West, John B. "Chapter 8: Respiratory Failure." In *Pulmonary Pathophysiology: The Essentials*, 7th ed. Baltimore: Lippincott Williams & Wilkins, a Wolters Kluwer business, 2008.

Figures

Figure 5.1: The inflammatory response of ARDS causes blockade of pulmonary vasculature. Rosen, Yale. 2010. CC BY-SA 2.0. From Flickr.

Figure 5.2: Pathophysiological events of ARDS. Grey, Kindred. 2022. CC BY 4.0. https://archive.org/details/5.3_20220203

Figure 5.3: Alveolar wall edema and onset of hyaline membrane formation during the exudative phase of ARDS. Rosen, Yale and Pillappa, Raghavendra. 2009. CC BY-SA 2.0. From Flickr.

Figure 5.4: Proliferation of type II cells and infiltration of fibroblasts in the proliferative phase of ARDS. Rosen, Yale and Pillappa, Raghavendra. 2009. CC BY-SA 2.0. From Flickr.

Figure 5.5: Fibrotic stage of ARDS. Rosen, Yale. 2010. CC BY-SA 2.0. From Flickr.

Figure 5.6: Pathophysiology of ARDS. Grey, Kindred. 2022. CC BY 4.0. https://archive.org/details/5.7_20220203

Figure 5.7: Diffuse bilateral densities associated with ARDS. Lorente, E., et al. 2020. CC BY-NC-SA 3.0. "Image 1" from https://doi.org/10.53347/rID-75182.

6. Lung Cancer

Learning objectives

- Describe the four major categories of primary lung cancer and the associated risk factors.
- Describe the clinical manifestations of lung cancer.

This chapter will deal with only primary lung cancer (i.e., that originating in the lung), although many other forms of cancer that originate outside of the lung commonly metastasize to the pulmonary system. By far the most common site of malignant neoplasm is the bronchial mucosa and so it is referred to as bronchogenic carcinoma. Most cases are related to smoking, and the risk of bronchogenic carcinoma is related to the duration and intensity of smoking—two packs a day for twenty years increases risk of lung cancer seventy times above a nonsmoker's risk. Other environmental or occupational factors can play a role, and when compounded with smoking the effect on risk can be multiplicative rather than additive, similar to asbestos exposure.

About half of neoplasms arise centrally, while the other half have a more peripheral origin in the smaller airways; but this is often very difficult to ascertain in advanced disease. The upper lobes are more commonly involved, particularly in the anterior segments, and the right lobe is more commonly involved than the left.

Four major types of bronchogenic carcinoma can be distinguished by histology, epidemiology, clinical features, and prognosis. They are:

1. squamous cell,
2. adenocarcinoma,
3. large cell, and
4. small cell.

Let us look at the features of each.

Squamous Cell

Squamous cell cancer accounts for about one-third of all lung cancers and is more common in men. It is pathologically characterized by keratin formation between cells and the development of large, well-outlined islands of cancer cells. It is usually centrally located and associated with the main bronchi. Metastasis tends to be local, affecting the surrounding areas and lymph nodes.

Adenocarcinoma

Adenocarcinoma also accounts for about one-third of cases but is the most common lung cancer in women. The lesion has a glandular structure and may produce mucin. This is usually a peripheral lesion and distant metastasis is common.

Large Cell

Large cell is less common and is seen in about 10 percent of cases, most of whom are male. The diagnosis is made by cell size, which is large and easily distinguished from squamous cell cancer or adenocarcinoma. The lesions can be anywhere in the lung but are often found in the periphery. This is a fast-growing cancer and so is frequently diagnosed at a later disease stage.

Small Cell

The previous three types of cancer are collectively known as non-small cell lung cancer. Alternatively, small cell cancer is found in about 15 percent of cases. It is less predominant in men, and incidence in women is rising. The small cells have an oat-like appearance, and the most common small cell cancer is known as oat cell carcinoma and the lesions frequently have endocrine function. Originating in the main bronchi this cancer spreads very quickly into other thoracic and extrathoracic sites, and this form carries a very poor prognosis.

The characteristics of these forms of lung cancer are summarized in table 6.1.

Squamous cell	**Adenocarcinoma**	**Large cell**	**Small cell**
~33% of cases	~33% of cases	~10% of cases	~10–15% of cases
More common in men	More common in women	Mostly found in men	Increasing rate in women
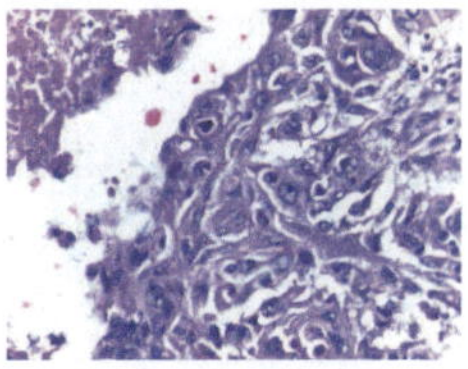	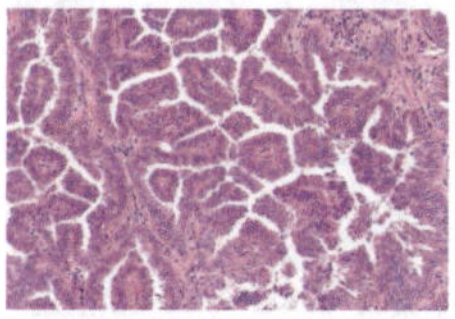	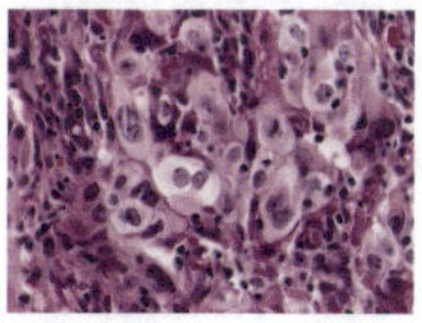	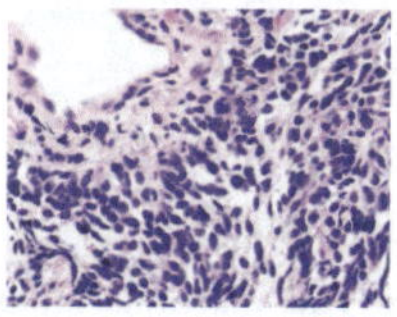
Keratin bridges between cells	Glandular architecture (may produce mucin)	Diagnosis made by size of cells	Oat-like appearance, endocrine function
Islands of cancer cells	Distant metastasis is common	Fast growing, often diagnosed as established disease	Highly malignant, rapid, and widespread metastasis
Most centrally located around main bronchi and affect local tissue	Frequently a peripheral lesion	Can be anywhere in the lung but more often peripheral	Starts in main bronchi but rapidly spreads

Table 6.1: Summary of forms of lung cancer.

Clinical Signs

The signs and symptoms can be variable and diverse depending on the location, type, size, and rapidity of growth. Patients may even be asymptomatic when the lesion is found on chest x-ray or with bronchoscope.

The most common symptom is cough, but unfortunately the patient, likely being a smoker, may be accustomed to cough and not think anything of it. Bloody sputum occurs in only about half of patients and is a frequent cause for them seeking medical advice, and severe hemoptysis is uncommon.

Chest pain is fairly common and ranges from a mild ache or feeling of heaviness, to severe and unremitting. Pain does not necessarily indicate pleural or chest wall involvement, although significant steady pain is more indicative of this complication.

Dyspnea may arise as the tumor obstructs a major airway or causes a large pleural effusion, but it can also be due to underlying bronchopulmonary disease.

Physical exam is likely to be normal in the early stages of the disease, but as the cancer progresses the exam usually reveals signs associated with either bronchial obstruction or a consequence of metastasis. Bronchial obstruction can lead to wheeze or other modified breath sounds, atelectasis, down-stream pneumonia, or pleural effusion. Paraneoplastic syndromes associated with the cancer can cause disruption to other systems and lead to characteristic weight loss, muscle wasting, and digital clubbing.

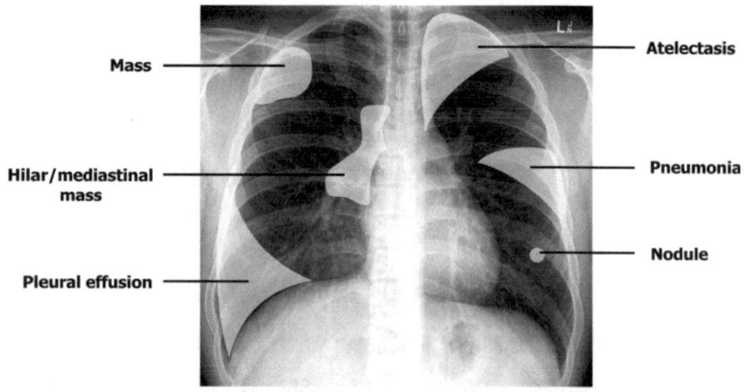

Figure 6.1: Potential radiographic findings in lung cancer.

Chest x-ray is usually only capable of detecting advanced cancer stages, and therefore is not the best screening tool. Low-dose CT screening can be used to detect early stages of disease before symptoms arise and is advised for patients between fifty to eighty years old with a twenty-pack-per-year smoking history or who have quit smoking in the past fifteen years. Once the disease is established, however, the x-ray's findings can either be direct detection of a mass, or a secondary consequence of the mass; therefore they are quite variable (figure 6.1).

- A mass may show as a solitary **nodule** or **coin lesion**, and peripheral lesions are most commonly associated with adenocarcinoma.
- Invasion of the tumor to lymph nodes may be observed as a **hilar** or **mediastinal mass** and is common with small cell carcinoma.
- Large cell cancer is frequently associated with **large peripheral masses** that may cavitate.
- Squamous cell carcinoma is frequently associated with bronchial obstruction, so as well as being detected as a mass it (and the other forms of cancer) can lead to detectable secondary effects such as atelectasis or a pneumonia that persistently appears in the same location. Pleural effusions, which can be massive, are sometimes the radiographic manifestation of lung cancer.
- Thoracic CT imaging is more useful for delineation of the original lesion and is now routinely used as a screening tool for current or ex-smokers.

References, Resources, and Further Reading

Text

Farzan, Sattar, with Doris L. Hunsinger and Mary L. Phillips. "Chapter 20." In *A Concise Handbook of Respiratory Diseases*. Reston, VA: Reston Publishing Company, 1978.

Husain, Aliya N. "Chapter 15: The Lung." In *Robbins and Cotran Pathologic Basis of Disease*, 9th ed., edited by Vinay Kumar, Abul K. Abbas, and John C. Aster. Philadelphia: Saunders, an imprint of Elsevier Inc., 2015.

Figures

Table 6.1: Summary of forms of lung cancer. Includes Squamous Cell Carcinoma Lung 40x by Calicut Medical College from WikimediaCommons (CC BY-SA 4.0), Papillary adenocarcinoma of the lung – intermed mag by Nephron from WikimediaCommons (CC BY-SA 3.0), Large cell carcinoma of the lung by The Armed Forces Institute of Pathology (AFIP) from WikimediaCommons (Public domain), and Lung small cell carcinoma (1) by core needle biopsy by KGH from WikimediaCommons (CC BY-SA 3.0).

Figure 6.1: Potential radiographic findings in lung cancer. Grey, Kindred. 2022. CC BY-NC-SA 3.0. Includes Normal frontal chest x-ray by Gaillard, F., et al. from https://doi.org/10.53347/rID-8090 (labels and shaded areas added) (CC BY-NC-SA 3.0). https://archive.org/details/6.2_20220203

7. Pulmonary Embolism

Learning objectives

- Describe the factors contributing to the occurrence of pulmonary embolism.
- Describe the pathophysiological consequences and clinical manifestations of pulmonary embolism.

Like any other embolism, an embolus affecting the lung tissue can be made of fat, amniotic fluid, tumor, tissue fragment, or foreign body, but by far the most common cause of pulmonary emboli are blood clots.

The lung contains the first diverging vascular network after the venous system so is particularly vulnerable to deep vein thrombi (DVT) breaking away, traveling through the progressively widening veins, through the right heart, and wedging into the progressively narrowing pulmonary arterial system.

Pathology of Pulmonary Embolism (PE)

About 90 percent of PEs are caused by deep vein thrombi, but at least one of three main predisposing factors (**Virchow's triad**) are present in a case of PE:

1. Abnormal vessel walls,
2. Stagnation of blood, and
3. Increased coagulability.

Abnormal vessel walls: Damage to the inner wall of veins causes adherence of blood platelets and activation of clotting factors. Similarly inflammation or trauma of the vein or surrounding area can lead to a risk of local clotting.

Venous stasis: Venous stasis appears to be the most important factor in thrombus formation, and cases of PE are often preceded by periods of immobility (top tip: a USMLE question with a long-haul flight in the stem should raise the PE flag). But other causes of disrupted venous blood flow can elevate the risk.

Hypercoagulability: Any condition that increases coagulability elevates the risk of PE, and most are due to trauma of some form or another or an elevated inflammatory state such as cancer or the postsurgery state. Birth control pills predispose the patient to thromboembolic disease so thereby also increase the risk of PE.

Pathophysiology of PE

The pathophysiology and clinical severity of PE depend on the number and size of the emboli, so clinical manifestations can be highly variable. In fact, PE is suspected to be much more common than previously thought because of improved detection techniques revealing more small and asymptomatic cases.

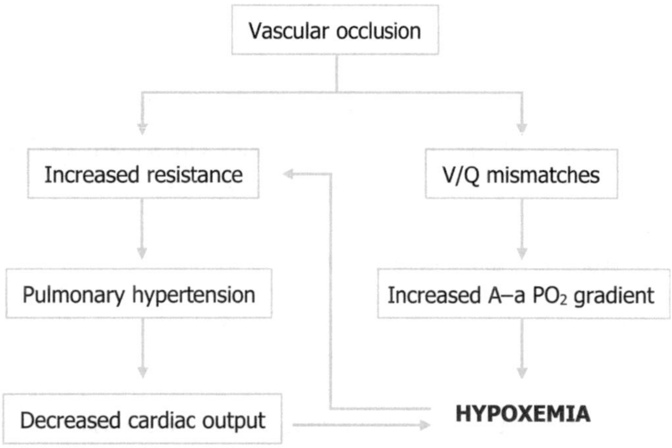

Figure 7.1: Pathophysiology of pulmonary embolism.

Small emboli that can travel further into the vasculature may cause occlusion of relatively small areas of the lung, but with these areas receiving no perfusion and still being ventilated V/Q becomes inappropriately high. Not being able to pass the occlusion, blood will be diverted to other areas of the lung, and consequently cause them to be overperfused, lowering V/Q.

Depending on the size and number of emboli, these V/Q mismatches can produce a widening **alveolar-arterial PO_2 difference** and lead to hypoxemia.

With larger emboli that occlude larger vessels there will not only be a larger impact on gas exchange, but also a more increase in pulmonary vascular resistance. The extreme (and thankfully rare) case is a "saddle" embolus that is large enough to straddle the bifurcation of the pulmonary trunk, obstruct the left and right pulmonary arteries, and lead to immediate hemodynamic collapse. In lesser cases, pulmonary hypertension will overwhelm the thin myocardium of the right ventricle, and as pulmonary arterial pressure approaches right ventricle pressure then cardiac output will fall. This will exaggerate the hypoxemia and cause the pulmonary vasculature to perform its normal vasoconstrictive response to low oxygen tensions that in turn worsens the pulmonary hypertension (summarized in figure 7.1).

Pulmonary infarction, however, is rare, occurring in only 10 percent of PE cases. The lung tissue is supplied by the bronchial circulation so can usually survive the embolism in the pulmonary circulation unless there is preexisting cardiac disease.

Clinical Signs of PE

The clinical manifestations of PE vary widely, from asymptomatic when emboli are small or few, to sudden death when they are large or numerous.

Signs of DVT may precede PE cases, such as leg pain, venous swelling, or warm skin over the thrombus site, but these are present in less than half of patients. Once instigated, the presenting symptom of PE is usually dyspnea but can also include chest pain. There can be clinical clues in the dyspnea as it has a rapid onset and is disproportionate to any initial clinical findings. The nature of its onset also tends to generate significant anxiety. Chest pain can start as anginal but then become more pleuritic.

Hemoptysis is less common but an important symptom. In severe cases involving massive PE tachypnea, tachycardia and cyanosis are usually present.

Because of the mechanical and metabolic strain on the heart, cardiac manifestations, including arrhythmia, acute cor pulmonale, or signs of cardiac failure or shock, may be detected with an increased difference between alveolar and arterial PO_2s.

The chest x-ray will appear normal, unless there are complications such as pleural effusion, atelectasis, or pulmonary infarction. CT angiography is used to detect the presence of a PE when suspicion is high. When suspicion is lower, labs will include a **D-dimer** test (a protein fragment produced by a dissolving clot), which, if negative, can help rule out the presence of a PE, but if positive would require further investigation (e.g., CT angiography) for confirmation.

References, Resources, and Further Reading

Text

Farzan, Sattar, with Doris L. Hunsinger and Mary L. Phillips. "Chapter 21." In A *Concise Handbook of Respiratory Diseases*. Reston, VA: Reston Publishing Company, 1978.

Husain, Aliya N. "Chapter 15: The Lung." In *Robbins and Cotran Pathologic Basis of Disease*, 9th ed., edited by Vinay Kumar, Abul K. Abbas, and John C. Aster. Philadelphia: Saunders, an imprint of Elsevier Inc., 2015.

West, John B. "Chapter 6: Vascular Diseases." In *Pulmonary Pathophysiology: The Essentials*, 7th ed. Baltimore: Lippincott Williams & Wilkins, a Wolters Kluwer business, 2008.

Figures

Figure 7.1: Pathophysiology of pulmonary embolism. Grey, Kindred. 2022. CC BY 4.0. https://archive.org/details/7.1_20220203

8. Immunological Diseases of the Lung

Learning objectives

- Compare and contrast the mechanisms and manifestations of hypersensitivity pneumonitis, Goodpasture's syndrome, systemic lupus erythematosus, rheumatoid disease, progressive systemic sclerosis, and polymyositis.

The lung is no different from any other organ in that it is susceptible to disorders of the immune system. One might argue that it is surprising that the lung does not encounter more problems, given the lung's exposure to the environment and the myriad antigens it encounters. Before we start looking at a few specific disorders, let us quickly review the four mechanisms through which the immune system might disrupt lung tissue.

A type 1 reaction, or **immediate hypersensitivity** (table 8.1), is a result of overexpression of IgE (table 8.1). When an antigen binds to the overexpressed IgE on the surface of mast cells, the cell releases histamine and leukotrienes that in turn induce an inappropriate or exaggerated inflammatory response. Allergic asthma is an example of a type 1 reaction.

A type 2 reaction, or **antibody-dependent cytotoxic reaction** (table 8.1), is the result of a circulating antibody reacting with a component of a cell or tissue. The formation of this inappropriate immune complex results in the cell or tissue being flagged for attack by the immune system. Goodpasture's syndrome is an example of a type 2 reaction.

A type 3 reaction, or **immune complex reaction** (table 8.1), is the result of an immune complex forming either locally or circulating from elsewhere and then depositing itself in tissue; the immune complex then instigates an immune system attack that involves the tissue. Pulmonary vasculitis can be caused by type 3 immune disorders.

Lastly, a type 4 reaction, or **cell-mediated hypersensitivity** (table 8.1), is caused by a population of hypersensitive T cells whose response to an antigen is exaggerated and leads to the proliferation of that cell population and the release of lymphokines to induce an inflammatory response. While this pattern is the same as the normal response to many infections, the magnitude of the response is inappropriate and can lead to pathological changes, such as allergic alveolitis.

Type of immune mechanism	Visual	Description
Type 1	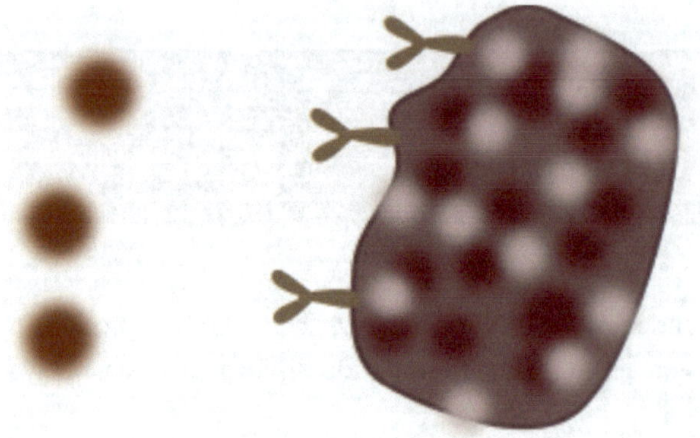	- Antigen-IgE interaction - Mast cell release of histamine, leukotrienes - E.g., allergic asthma
Type 2	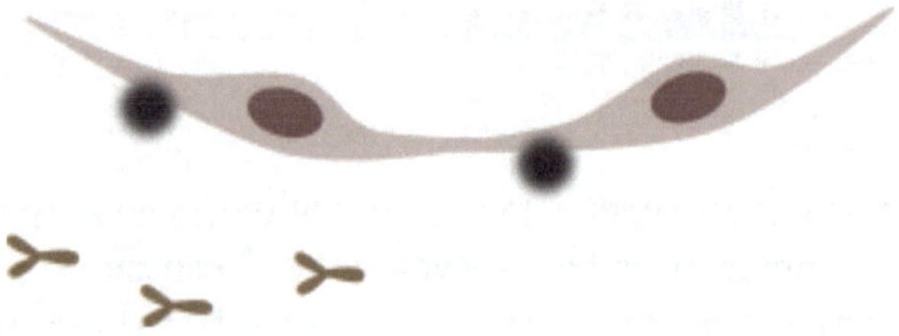	- Component of cell acts as antigen - Antibodies bind and cell attacked - E.g., Goodpasture's syndrome
Type 3	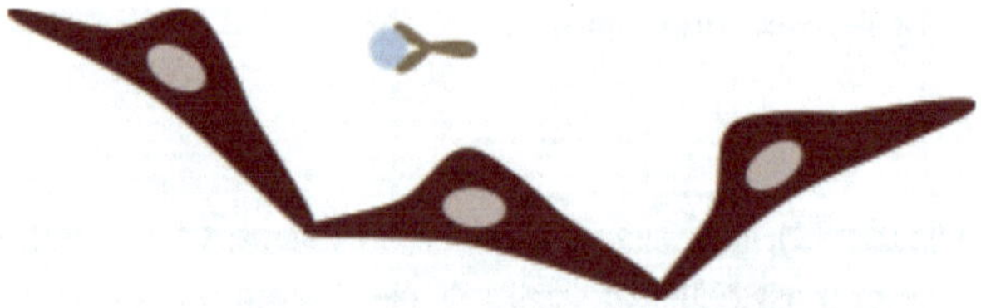	- A remotely or locally formed immune complex embeds into tissue - E.g., pulmonary vasculitis
Type 4	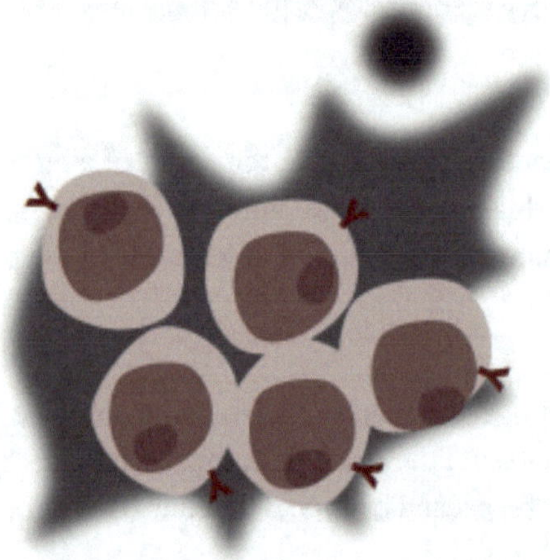	- A sensitized T-lymphocyte responds to arrival of an antigen with proliferation and release of lymphokines - E.g., allergic alveolitis

Table 8.1: Types of immune mechanisms involved in lung tissue injury.

With those mechanisms defined, let us look at some specific disorders.

Hypersensitivity Pneumonitis

Also called **extrinsic allergic alveolitis**, **hypersensitivity pneumonitis** is usually initiated by inhaled particles that are small enough to reach the alveoli and act as antigens to induce an immune response. There are many different types of particle that can be involved. The type of particle or the occupation in which the exposure occurs frequently gives its name to the condition it causes, for example farmer's lung occurs after exposure to moldy hay and the antigen *Micropolyspora foeni*, bird breeder's lung occurs with exposure to avian proteins, cheese worker's lung occurs after inhalation and sensitization to moldy cheese. The list goes on, but the pathogenetic mechanisms are the same and the pathological/radiographic findings are indistinguishable, meaning all these diseases are considered part of the same syndrome.The time line of exposure to manifestation of symptoms, the measured serum antibody titers, and the demonstration of antibodies and inflammatory changes in the lung suggest hypersensitivity pneumonitis includes both type 3 and type 4 reactions (table 8.1).

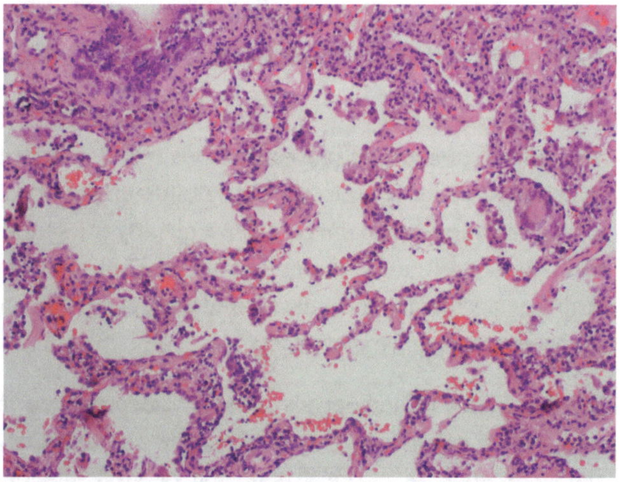

Figure 8.1: Acute phase of hypersensitivity pneumonitis. Note presence of giant cells in the alveolar septum on the center, right-hand side of field of view.

In the acute phase, lymphocytes and macrophages infiltrate the alveolar walls and loose granulomas can form. The presence of multi-nucleated giant cells (figure 8.2), are helpful in diagnosis, but more typical is a dramatic rise in lymphocyte count in BAL fluid, particularly CD8+ cells.

In the subacute phase there is evidence of interstitial thickening and the onset of fibrosis can be seen. Involvement of the bronchioles is seen with evidence of chronic bronchiolitis. The chronic form is marked by significant fibrosis (figure 8.3), to the extent it is indistinguishable from pulmonary fibrosis with distinctive fibrotic patterns and all the hallmarks of restrictive lung disease.

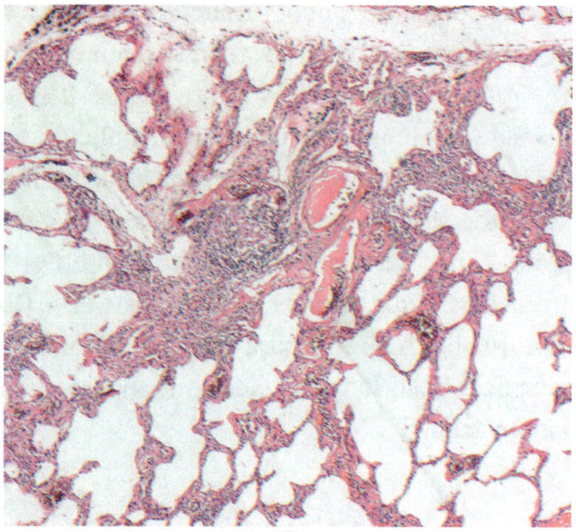

(C)

Figure 8.2: Chronic phase of hypersensitivity pneumonitis with established fibrosis.

Clinical signs

How hypersensitivity pneumonitis presents is somewhat dependent on the form of exposure the patient had.

With brief but heavy exposure, an acute presentation of pneumonitis will present with fever, malaise, cough, and dyspnea. Physical exam confirms the fever and tachypnea and cyanosis can reflect the severity of the response. Bibasilar rales are often present, but unless a type 1 hypersensitivity arises then wheeze is usually absent (but you might note here that concurrent allergenic asthma is not beyond the realms of possibility). This acute form usually resolves within a couple of days, but can reoccur when the patient is exposed to the causal agent again.

When exposure is light but prolonged, the onset of hypersensitivity pneumonitis is more insidious and clinically challenging. The patient will describe a slowly progressive cough and developing dyspnea, also weakness and weight loss. This form of onset is common with continuous exposure to organic dust. With this longer time line the patient is not usually aware of the symptom's relation to occupation and exposure persists until diffuse pulmonary fibrosis is established. At this point the signs and symptoms are related to respiratory insufficiency.

Goodpasture's Syndrome

The only pulmonary disease caused by a type 2 mechanism is Goodpasture's syndrome, which usually affects young males. It is caused by a circulating autoimmune antibody against Type IV collagen in the basement membranes of the alveoli and the renal glomeruli. Consequently the syndrome manifests as both renal and pulmonary dysfunction. The formation of an immune complex when the antibody binds to protein in the basement membrane initiates an immune response against the local tissue, and the main pulmonary manifestation is periodic **hemoptysis** caused by degradation of the alveolarcapillary interface.

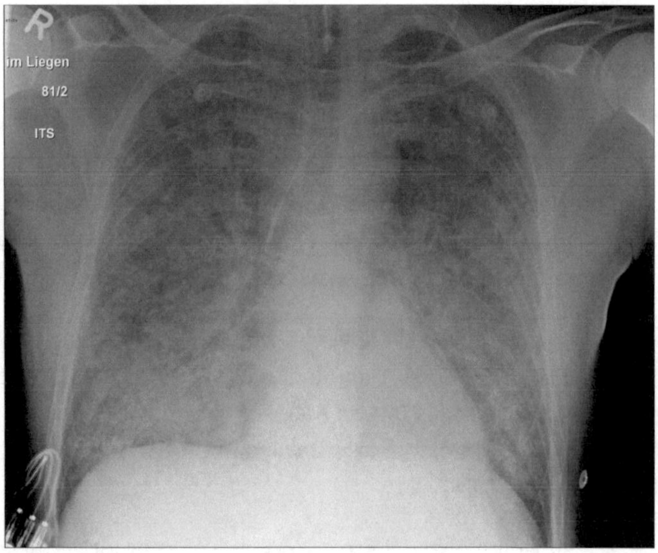

Figure 8.3: Patchy airspace consolidation associated with Goodpasture's syndrome.

The frequency of hemoptysis somewhat depends on the presence of other factors that affect the permeability of the lung, such as cigarette smoking or viral infection. Other manifestations include dyspnea, anemia, diffuse pulmonary infiltrate, and signs of kidney damage (hematuria as the glomerular basement membranes lose integrity).

The dyspnea no doubt occurs because of the patchy airspace consolidation that can be seen on chest x-ray as the diffuse pulmonary infiltrate (figure 8.3). In a severe episode, such as shown in this example, the patient may be hypoxic; however, distribution is often more patchy. Over the next several days the infiltrate clears but can leave a reticular pattern denoting a fibrotic reaction. Ironically, if lung transfer factor is tested the DLCO can be abnormally high because of the hemoglobin in the airspaces absorbing the carbon monoxide. The prognosis is poor with the patient usually succumbing to progressive kidney failure.

Systemic Diseases Affecting the Lung

Systemic Lupus Erythematosus (SLE)

Lupus erythematosus is a type 3 reaction. Autoantibodies are formed against cell components, particularly the nucleus and its associated proteins. The most common antibodies found are against single- or double-stranded DNA. About 70 percent of SLE patients have lung involvement that can be either acute or chronic.

Acute SLE

The acute form is referred to as lupus pneumonitis, and its signs and symptoms mimic bacterial pneumonia. It can have a rapidly progressive course with acute pleuritic chest pain and can lead to respiratory failure. The inflammation it involves can disrupt pulmonary capillaries and lead to hemorrhage. Patients with SLE are highly susceptible to infection, so diagnosis of an SLE patient should distinguish between respiratory tract infection and changes directly related to lupus. Changes in lupus come as flares followed by remission, and there are a number of triggers for flares including:

- drugs such as tetracycline and penicillin,
- viral infection, and
- exhaustion or emotional stress.

Chronic SLE

The chronic form can progress insidiously with no symptoms or physical findings, and so it frequently it goes unrecognized until later stages of the disease. The later stages are marked with the appearance of progressive fibrosis. This is evident in the chest x-rays in figure 8.4 showing the appearance of diffuse fibrosis over a twenty-month period in a young SLE patient. The fibrosis produces reduced lung volumes and basilar atelectasis may also occur. The increased recoil of the lung can also produce an elevated and weakened diaphragm. There may also be pleural involvement with effusions arising that are normally bilateral and small.

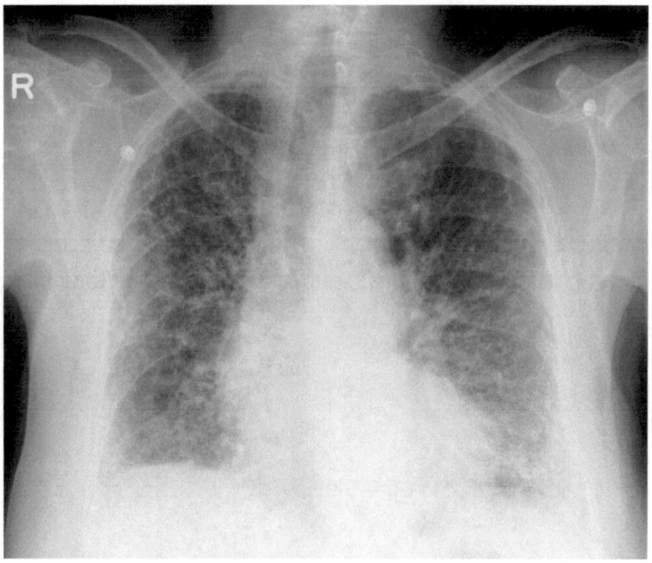

Figure 8.4: Progression of diffuse fibrosis in chronic SLE.

Rheumatoid Disease

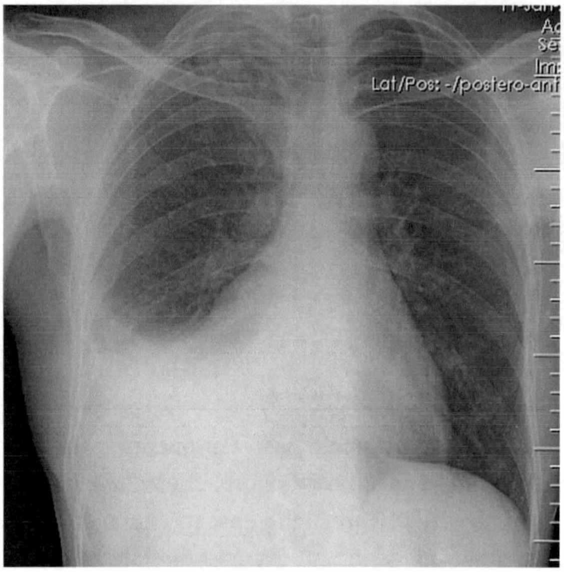

Figure 8.5: Pleural effusion in a rheumatoid patient.

More famous for its effect on the joints, rheumatoid disease can also affect the lungs and pleura. Rheumatoid factors that generate rheumatoid disease continue to be investigated, but in brief, they are antibodies generated against gamma globulins. Pleural and pulmonary lesions are probably the result of local immune complex-mediated reactions associated with high levels of circulating rheumatoid factors.

Up to 50 percent of rheumatoid patients show pulmonary or pleural manifestations, with pleural involvement being more common and most frequently manifested as pleural effusion (figure 8.5). The effusate tends to have low glucose, and this finding is useful for diagnosis. Pleural and pulmonary manifestations of rheumatoid disease are more common in male patients.

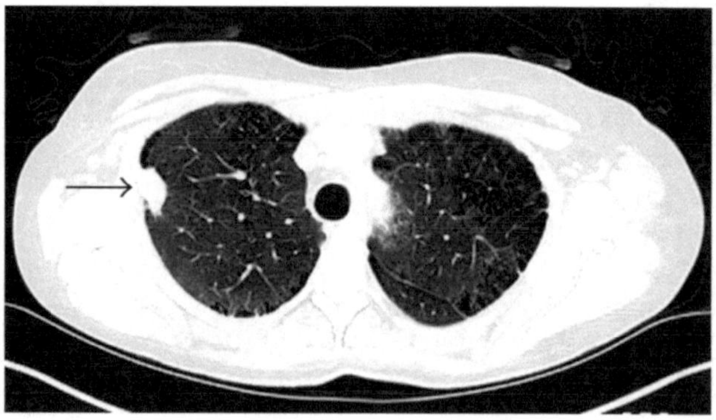

Figure 8.6: A nodular lesion (arrow) associated with rheumatoid disease.

Pulmonary involvement shows as either diffuse or nodular lesions (figure 8.6). The diffuse lesions are similar to those seen in idiopathic pulmonary fibrosis. The nodular lesions are variable in size and number and usually do not cause symptoms. They are known as **necrobiotic nodules** and are capable of cavitating. **Bronchiolitis obliterans organizing pneumonia** and **bronchiectasis** have also been seen in rheumatoid disease.

It should be noted here that some drugs used to treat difficult rheumatoid arthritis, such as gold preparations, methotrexate, and penicillamine, are toxic to the lung and can produce their own pulmonary lesions.

Progressive Systemic Sclerosis

Also known as scleroderma, progressive systemic sclerosis primarily affects the blood vessels and connective tissue and likely has an autoimmune mechanism. The result is dysregulation of fibroblasts and uncontrolled collagen formation. The disease can affect many organs and tissues, and pulmonary manifestations are common.

The most common pulmonary findings are interstitial fibrosis, bronchiolar dilation, and pleural fibrosis, as well as the vascular changes that are seen in other organs. These changes produce dyspnea, cough, and basilar rales. The vascular changes can produce pulmonary hypertension that may lead to **cor pulmonale**.

The radiographic findings are similar to pulmonary fibrosis with the early stage of the disease showing fine reticular patterning that progresses to honeycombing in the late stage of the disease (figure 8.7). These changes are mostly found in the lower lung fields. As you might expect, the disease has restrictive characteristics along with diffusion abnormalities that produce hypoxemia during exercise.

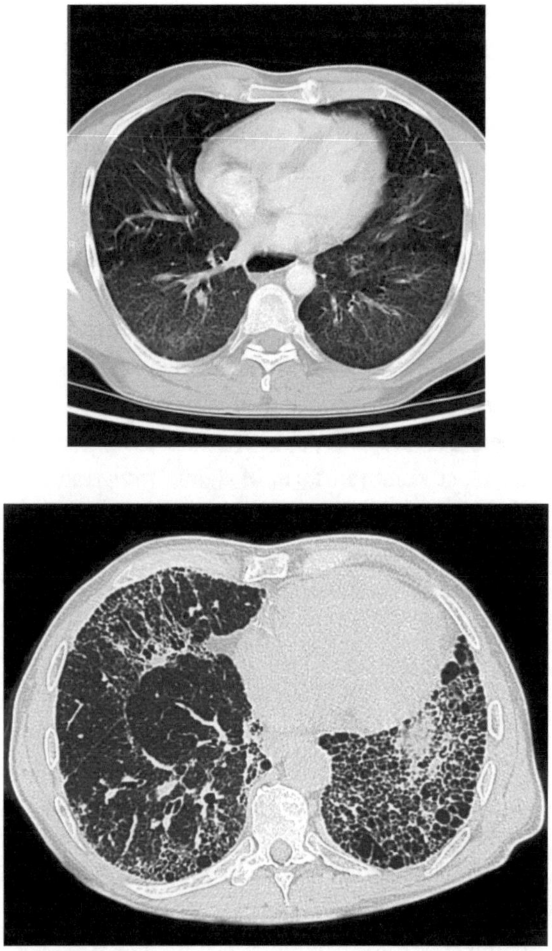

Figure 8.7: Fine reticular fibrosis in lower lung fields (upper CT image) progressing to honeycombing (lower CT image).

Polymyositis

Polymyositis is an autoimmune disease that attacks striated muscle through a cell-mediated mechanism, but can also affect other organ systems, including the lung.

There is some direct involvement with development of bronchiolitis obliterans organizing pneumonia (BOOP) and chronic interstitial pneumonitis and fibrosis. But the most frequent respiratory complications are a result of the respiratory muscles and muscles involved with swallowing becoming affected. Poor control of swallowing and inability to generate effective cough promote aspiration and retention of airway secretions. This is a recipe for bronchopneumonia—and this ends up being the most common form of death. Infection risk is often increased by the patient taking large doses of corticosteroids or immunosuppressive drugs to address the disease.

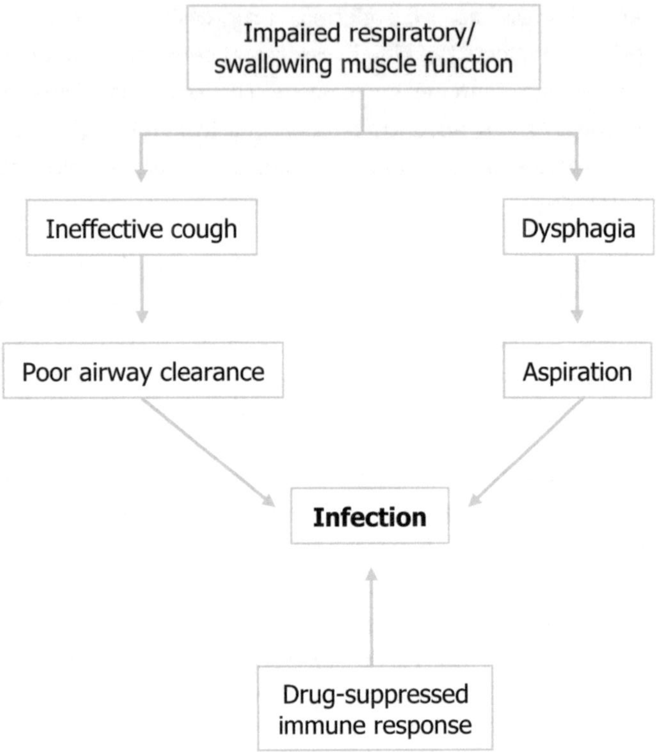

Figure 8.8: The pathophysiological sequence for the most common cause of death in polymyositis.

Summary

To summarize, the immunological responses to inhaled particles, localized immune responses, and systemic immunological disease can produce pulmonary manifestations that are generally related to acute and then chronic inflammatory responses. The distinguishing features and pulmonary manifestations are summarized in table 8.2.

Disorder	Immunological response	Pulmonary manifestations	Distinguishing/associated features
Hypersensitivity pneumonitis	Type 3 and 4	Fibrosis	Early presence of giant cells
Goodpasture's syndrome	Type 2	- Hemoptysis - Airspace consolidation	- Associated renal disease - Potentially high DLCO
SLE	Type 3	- Acute: pneumonia-like - Chronic: fibrosis	- Multiple organ involvement - Butterfly rash on face
Rheumatoid disease	Type 3	Nodular lesions	Skeletal/joint involvement
Sclerosis	Type 3	Interstitial and pleural fibrosis	Associated vascular involvement
Polymyositis	Type 4	Respiratory muscle weakness	Inflammatory infiltration of skeletal muscle

Table 8.2: Summary of immune and systemic disorders that affect the lung.

References, Resources, and Further Reading

Text

Farzan, Sattar, with Doris L. Hunsinger and Mary L. Phillips. "Chapters 13–14." In A *Concise Handbook of Respiratory Diseases*. Reston, VA: Reston Publishing Company, 1978.

Husain, Aliya N. "Chapter 15: The Lung." In *Robbins and Cotran Pathologic Basis of Disease*, 9th ed., edited by Vinay Kumar, Abul K. Abbas, and John C. Aster. Philadelphia: Saunders, an imprint of Elsevier Inc., 2015.

Figures

Table 8.1: Types of immune mechanisms involved in lung tissue injury. Includes Immune mechanism – type 1 by Kindred Grey from Internet archive (CC BY 4.0), Immune mechanism – type 2 by Kindred Grey from Internet archive (CC BY 4.0), Immune mechanism – type 3 by Kindred Grey from Internet archive (CC BY 4.0), and Immune mechanism – type 4 by Kindred Grey from Internet archive (CC BY 4.0).Figure 8.1: Acute phase of hypersensitivity pneumonitis. Mutleysmith. 2012. CC BY-SA 3.0. From WikimediaCommons.

Figure 8.2: Chronic phase of hypersensitivity pneumonitis with established fibrosis. Kouranos, Vasileios, Joseph Jacob, Andrew Nicholson, and Elizabetta Renzoni. 2017. CC BY 4.0. Figure 3C from mdpi.

Figure 8.3: Patchy airspace consolidation associated with Goodpasture's syndrome. Krzys617. 2016. CC BY-SA 3.0. From Wikidoc.

Figure 8.4: Progression of diffuse fibrosis in chronic SLE. Bickle, I., et al. 2016. CC BY-NC-SA 3.0. From https://doi.org/10.53347/rID-46209.

Figure 8.5: Pleural effusion in a 52-year old male rheumatoid patient. Pai, V., et al. 2014. CC BY-NC-SA 3.0. From https://doi.org/10.53347/rID-27112.

Figure 8.6: A nodular lesion (arrow) associated with rheumatoid disease. Chhakchhuak, Christine L., Mehdi Khosravi, and Kristine M. Lohr. 2013. CC BY 4.0. From Hindawi.

Figure 8.7: Fine reticular fibrosis in lower lung fields (upper CT image) progressing to honeycombing (lower CT image). Includes case 3 by Yang, N., Sharma, R., et al. from https://doi.org/10.53347/rID-8608 (CC BY-NC-SA 3.0) and image 1 by Gaillard, F., et al. from https://doi.org/10.53347/rID-35820 (CC BY-NC-SA 3.0).

Figure 8.8: The pathophysiological sequence for the most common cause of death in polymyositis. Grey, Kindred. 2022. CC BY 4.0. https://archive.org/details/8.9_20220203

9. Pleural Diseases

Learning objectives

- Distinguish the pathogenesis, pathophysiology, and clinical manifestations of pleural effusion, pleurisy, and pneumothorax.
- Relate the pathophysiology of pleural effusion and pneumothorax to lung and cardiac function.

While there are a few primary disorders of the pleura, their anatomy and location can make them susceptible to secondary diseases. The pleura fundamentally form a subatmospheric cavity within the thorax, making them susceptible to disorders that result in fluid accumulation (for example, cardiac failure). Conversely, the proximity of the pleura to other organs can mean pleural disease can affect other organs such as mediastinal structures and subdiaphragmatic viscera.

We will look at the most important and frequently occurring disorders of the pleura, namely:

- pleurisy,
- pleural effusion,
- pleural empyema, and
- pneumothorax.

To get warmed up, let us start with the simplest one, pleurisy.

Pleurisy

Pleurisy is synonymous with pleuritis and refers to inflammation of the pleural membranes that may be accompanied by pleural exudate or may remain "dry." Inflammation of the membranes may be mild and transient due to common conditions such as bacterial or viral infection, or it may be severe and chronic and indicative of more serious conditions, such as lupus and rheumatoid arthritis.

The inflammation causes thickening of the membranes that may cause them to impinge on the pleural space. Prolonged inflammation leads to an accumulation of pleural macrophages, and these in turn initiate a proliferation of fibrocytes. The inflammatory process may prevent the membranes from moving freely, and in some patients the two inflamed membranes sliding against each other can produce an audible pleural friction rub, which sounds like leather rubbing against leather or walking on fresh snow. The hallmark symptom of a pleural rub is sudden onset chest pain associated with inhalation and cough.

In prolonged pathological conditions, the membranes may adhere, and calcium deposits can appear in old pleural fibrosis and are often associated with chronic conditions such as asbestosis. When significant, this level of fibrosis may restrict respiratory movement.

Pleural Effusion

In our description of pleurisy we eluded to our next pleural disorder, **pleural effusion**. The normally small amount of pleural fluid is sufficient to lubricate the movement of the lungs and is not detectable on x-ray without specialized radiography. Pleural effusion is the abnormal accumulation of fluid in the pleural space and is easily detectable. As with the formation of fluid accumulation in any part of the body, a normal fluid level in the pleural space is dependent on a balanced rate of formation and reabsorption. In pleural effusion, this balance is lost.

Initially it was thought that pleural fluid was formed by hydrostatic pressure in capillaries in the parietal membrane pushing fluid into the pleural space, and the fluid was then absorbed by capillaries in the visceral membrane. However, there is mounting evidence to show that reabsorption is actually performed by the lymph vessels in the parietal membrane. The low hydrostatic pressure and large capacity of these vessels helps maintain the normal, small volume of pleural fluid. Pleural effusion can be caused by:

1. too much fluid formation,
2. too little fluid absorption, or
3. a combination of both.

For example, pleural effusion in cardiac pulmonary edema occurs as fluid leaks across the visceral pleura from the lung.

Two broad classifications exist, transudate and exudate, so let us compare them now (summary in table 9.1).

Transudative effusion occurs when there is a disturbance in the Starling's forces influencing fluid movement across the capillary. As such transudate can be caused by an increase in hydrostatic force pushing fluid out of the capillary, such as in congestive heart failure, or a decrease in the plasma oncotic pressure retaining fluid in the capillary, such as in kidney or liver disease. This results in a transudate with low specific gravity, protein concentration, and cell count.

Exudative effusion is caused by increased capillary permeability, such as that caused by the inflammatory process. Relate this back to your understanding of exudative pleurisy (figure 9.1). As larger molecules can exit the leaky capillaries, exudative effusion has a higher specific gravity, higher protein concentration, and likely a higher cell count.

Transudate	**Exudate**
Increased hydrostatic pressure	Increased capillary permeability
Decreased plasma oncotic pressure	
- Low specific gravity - Low protein concentration - Low cell count	- Higher specific gravity - Higher protein concentration - Increased cell count

Table 9.1: Comparison of transudative and exudative pleural effusions.

The manifestation of pleural effusion varies with the quantity of fluid accumulation and the time line. Symptoms may in fact be absent when the effusion is small. In the case of exudative pleurisy, an initial rub pain may disappear as exudate accumulates and separates the rubbing pleural surfaces.

As the effusion volume increases the patient is likely to experience dyspnea and physical exam will more likely include dullness to percussion and absence of breath sounds as the effusion forms a fluid pillow around the lung.

As the severity of the effusion increases the patient will be severely short of breath, and the risk of the effusion pushing mediastinal structures to the contralateral side becomes significant and urgent (figure 9.1) as even mild displacement of the mediastinum can reduce cardiac output and produce hypotension. More significant displacement can become life threatening.

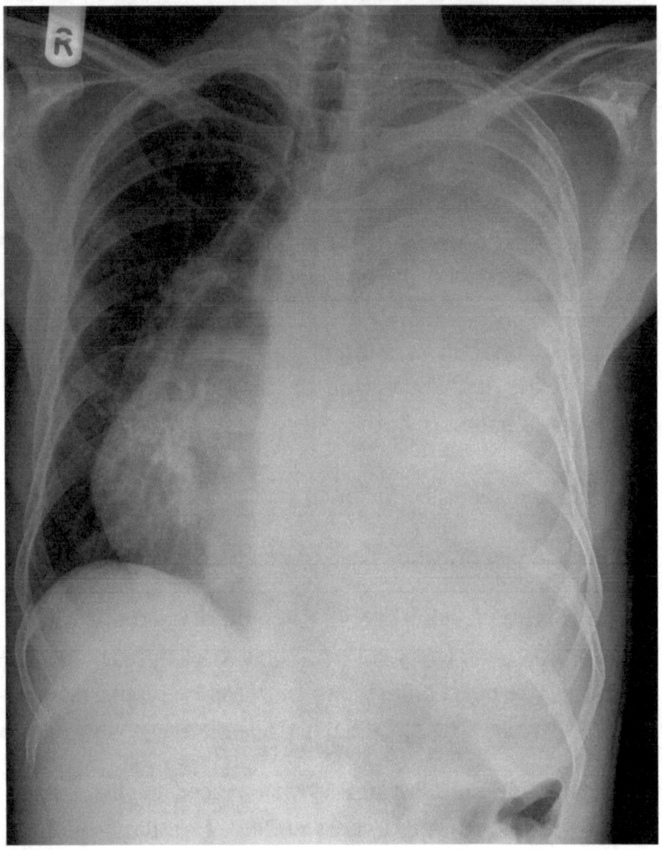

Figure 9.1: Severe pleural effusion leading to displacement of the mediastinum and heart to the right. This patient's condition is critical because of the threat to cardiac output.

As we have already mentioned, the pleural fluid's composition can provide a great deal of information about the underlying mechanism. We have already mentioned the ability to distinguish between an exudate and a transudate by analysis of the fluid. But gross inspection of the fluid can be revealing before lab tests are ready.

Fluid drawn through thoracentesis that appears clear and straw colored (figure 9.2) is likely to be transudate. The clarity of the fluid relates to a low protein content reflecting intact capillaries, and you should be looking for disturbances in Starling's forces. Lab results can confirm the integrity of the capillary beds. Clinically the pleural fluid's protein content and lactate dehydrogenase concentration are used and are expressed as a ratio with the patient's plasma concentrations. **Light's criteria** set diagnostic thresholds for these ratios to determine transudative or exudative effusions.

The higher protein of exudative effusion gives the fluid a more turbid or cloudy appearance, and high protein content may even give the fluid a foamy head (figure 9.2). Further lab analysis of the composition and cell content of the exudate can help determine the underlying cause of the leak. For example, presence of polymorphonuclear leukocytes is highly suggestive of pyrogenic infection, whereas predominance of lymphocytes is indicative of TB or malignancy.

Presence of lysed red blood cells will give the fluid a red turbid appearance (figure 9.2) and is indicative of trauma or malignancy, and again will require further investigation. If a malignancy has penetrated the lymphatics, such as the thoracic duct, the resultant chylous exudate will have a milky appearance.

A purulent fluid (figure 9.2) is indicative of infection within the pleural space and culturing the fluid will allow the pathogen to be determined. When pleural fluid is grossly purulent or contains pyogenic organisms we refer to this as **pleural empyema**. The most common route of entry for organisms is from underlying pneumonia or lung abscess, or through penetrative surgery or chest wound. The patient usually presents with fever and other manifestations of bacterial infection.

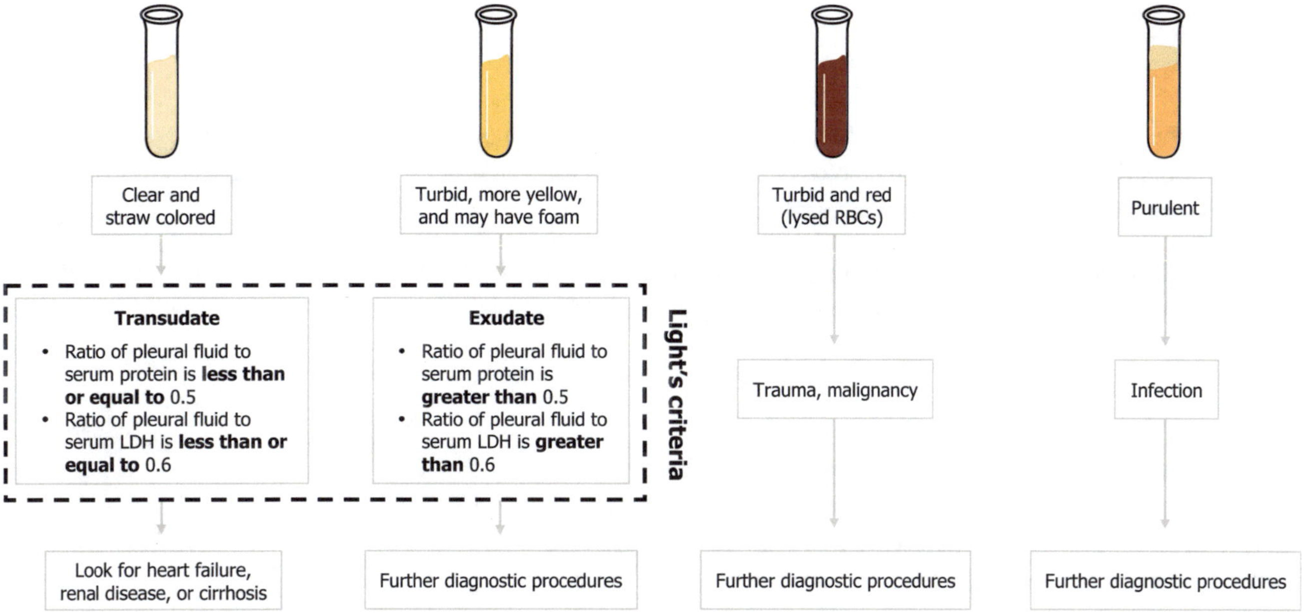

Figure 9.2: Appearance of pleural fluid and diagnosis.

Pneumothorax

Normally the negative pressure inside the pleural space opposes the lung's recoil and holds the lung surface to the interior of the thorax. If the pleural membranes are disrupted this subatmospheric or negative pressure is lost and the lung can recoil, or collapse. This is a pneumothorax.

The causal events of losing the negative pleural pressure divide pneumothoraces into one of two categories: spontaneous or traumatic. (A third category exists, artificial pneumothorax, which was intentionally induced as part of procedures that are very rarely used today.)

Spontaneous pneumothorax occurs in the absence of accidental or intentional trauma. When it occurs in otherwise healthy individuals it is usually the fault of anatomy and occurs mostly in tall, thin individuals with a long and narrow chest. If you compare the two body morphs in figure 9.3, the tall, thin torso has a lot of lung mass hanging below a relatively small apical section of pleural membrane compared to the other torso.

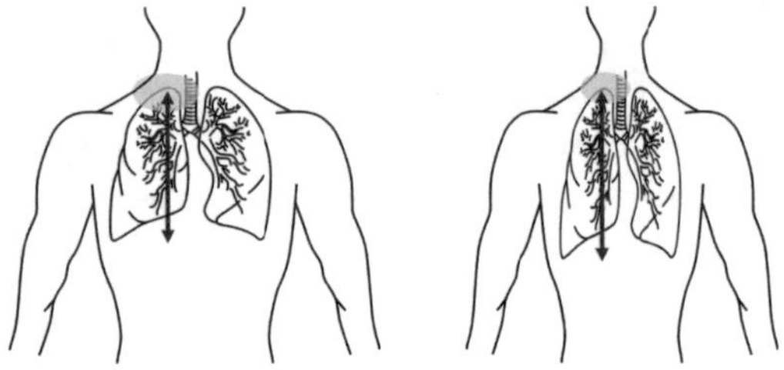

Figure 9.3: A tall, thin body morph (right) is more prone to a spontaneous pneumothorax.

The proportionately greater weight of lung per unit surface area at the apex increases the risk that bulla form (figure 9.4), then rupture causing loss of pleural membrane adhesion.

The most common cause of spontaneous pneumothorax in pulmonary patients is a ruptured bleb or bulla. These thin-walled, air-filled cavities are found near the pleural surface, particularly in cases of emphysema. In the past, TB was thought to be the most common cause of pneumothorax as its destructive path encroached on the pleural space.

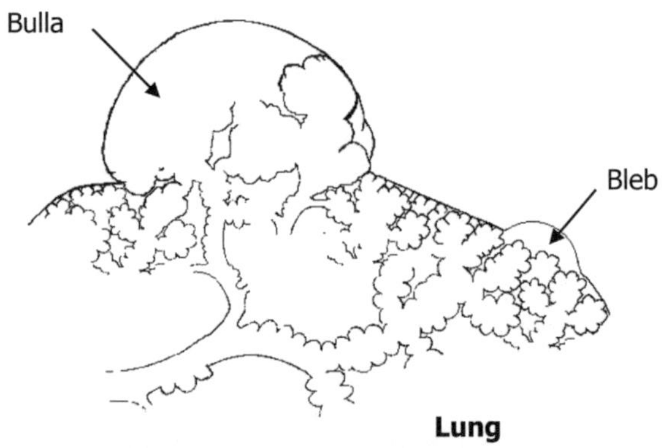

Traumatic pneumothorax is often a consequence of chest injury that involves laceration of the pleura. This might be due to a broken rib or penetrative wound to the chest that allows air to enter the pleural space and equilibrate with the atmosphere. The injury might not be malicious though as some procedures might inadvertently or unavoidably perforate the pleura, such as **thoracentesis**, pleural biopsy, lung biopsy, or subclavian vein puncture. Trauma from within the lung may also occur. Similar to the mechanism of a rupturing bleb, if excessive airway pressures are used during mechanical ventilation there is the risk that airspaces are disrupted and barotrauma involves the visceral pleura.

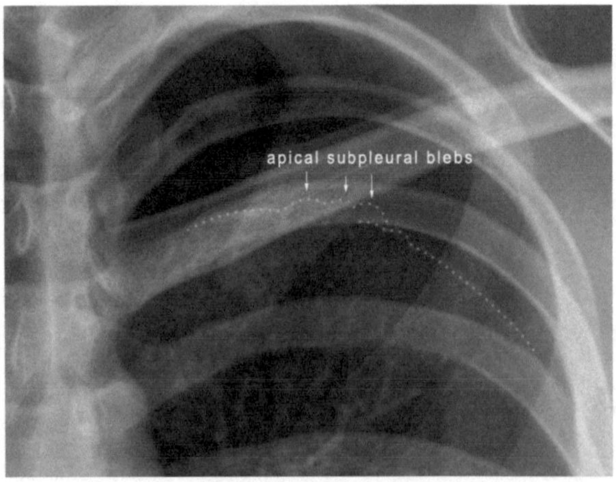

Figure 9.4: Rupturing bulla and blebs can lead to spontaneous pneumothorax.

The pneumothorax is readily identified with translucency on the affected side. The pathophysiology of a pneumothorax (figure 9.5) leads to hypoxia and hypercapnia in the affected lung through changes in perfusion and ventilation. Perfusion to the affected side is markedly reduced as the vasoconstrictive response to local hypoxia and the loss of radial traction to vessels profoundly increases vascular resistance. Consequently, perfusion shifts to the contralateral and unaffected lung. Similarly ventilation to the collapsed lung is minimal as airspaces are collapsed and airway resistance is very high, but the chemoreceptive reflexes increase ventilation to the unaffected lung where resistance is normal. Because perfusion and ventilation are shifted to the normal lung, V/Q mismatching may be compensated to some degree and severe hypoxemia may be avoided. When pneumothorax occurs patients usually describe a rapid onset of dyspnea and initial sudden sharp pain. The pain often then transitions into a dull ache.

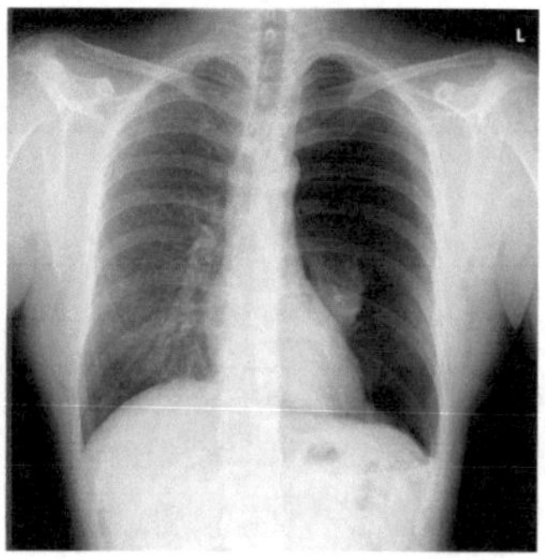

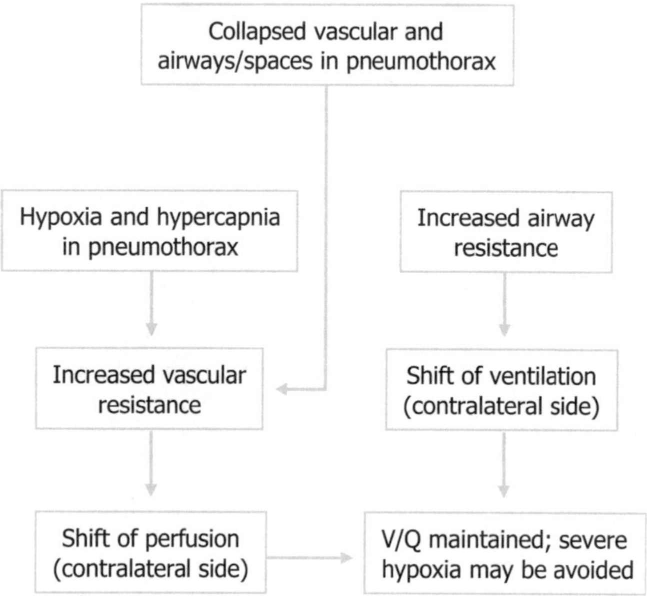

Figure 9.5: Pathophysiology of a pneumothorax

Tension pneumothorax may arise if the disruption to the pleural is such that the injury acts like a valve. During inspiration when thoracic pressure falls air enters the airways and also the thoracic cavity via the injury. During expiration when the thoracic pressure increases, the wound closes, stopping the air that entered the thoracic cavity from leaving. So with each inspiration more air enters while little or none leaves during the subsequent expiration. The accumulating volume can begin to push the heart and mediastinum to the contralateral side. This may severely affect cardiac output and rapidly become life threatening.

These CT scans in figure 9.6 shows a spontaneous pneumothorax (left panel) and a tension pneumothorax (right panel) with significant shift of the mediastinum over the contralateral hemithorax. So now you should be able to distinguish between the causes and mechanisms of these pleural disorders and determine their effects on pulmonary and cardiac function.

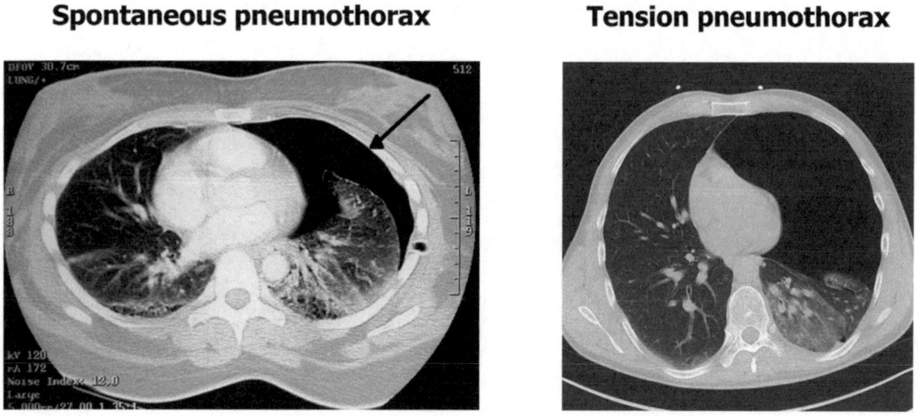

Figure 9.6: CT comparison of an uncomplicated pneumothorax and a tension pneumothorax.

References, Resources, and Further Reading

Text

Farzan, Sattar, with Doris L. Hunsinger and Mary L. Phillips. "Chapter 22." In A *Concise Handbook of Respiratory Diseases*. Reston, VA: Reston Publishing Company, 1978.

Husain, Aliya N. "Chapter 15: The Lung." In *Robbins and Cotran Pathologic Basis of Disease*, 9th ed., edited by Vinay Kumar, Abul K. Abbas, and John C. Aster. Philadelphia: Saunders, an imprint of Elsevier Inc., 2015.

West, John B. "Chapter 5: Restrictive Diseases." In *Pulmonary Pathophysiology: The Essentials*, 7th ed. Baltimore: Lippincott Williams & Wilkins, a Wolters Kluwer business, 2008.

Figures

Figure 9.1: Severe pleural effusion leading to mild displacement of the mediastinum. Bickle, I., et al. 2017. CC BY-NC-SA 3.0. From https://doi.org/10.53347/rID-56506.

Figure 9.2: Appearance of pleural fluid and diagnosis. Grey, Kindred. 2022. CC BY 4.0. Added Test Tube by Victoria Codes from Noun Project (added color)(CC BY 3.0). https://archive.org/details/9.3_20220203

Figure 9.3: A tall thin body morph (right) is more prone to a spontaneous pneumothorax. Grey, Kindred. 2022. CC BY 4.0. Added Lungs by iconmu from Noun Project (CC BY 3.0). https://archive.org/details/9.4_20220203

Figure 9.4: Rupturing bulla and blebs can lead to spontaneous pneumothorax. Grey, Kindred. 2022. Includes Pneumot rax bullae by Robertolyra from WikimediaCommons (public domain) and JZTg XeWvwrS45Dzl7SoSg288930 by Travis from Wikiradiography/MediaWiki (CC BY-SA 3.0). https://archive.org/details/9.5-new

Figure 9.5: Pathophysiology of a pneumothorax. Grey, Kindred. 2022. CC BY-NC-SA 3.0. Added case 1 by Gorrochategui, M., Niknejad, M., et al. from https://doi.org/10.53347/rID-4578 (CC BY-NC-SA 3.0). https://archive.org/details/9.6-real

Figure 9.6: CT comparison of an uncomplicated pneumothorax and a tension pneumothorax. Grey, Kindred. 2022. CC BY-NC-SA 3.0. Includes Pneumothorax CT by Doc James from WikimediaCommons (CC BY-SA 2.5) and image 1 by Wichmann, J., et al. from https://doi.org/10.53347/rID-25861 (CC BY-NC-SA 3.0). https://archive.org/details/9.6_20220203